American
Medical
Association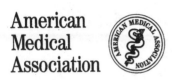

Guide to
Talking to Your Doctor

Other books by the American Medical Association

American Medical Association
Complete Guide to Men's Health

American Medical Association
Guide to Home Caregiving

American Medical Association
Family Medical Guide

American Medical Association
Complete Guide to Women's Health

American Medical Association
Complete Guide to Your Children's Health

American Medical Association
Family Health Cookbook

American Medical Association
Guide to Your Family's Symptoms

American Medical Association
Handbook of First Aid and Emergency Care

American Medical Association
Essential Guide to Menopause

American Medical Association
Essential Guide to Hypertension

American
Medical
Association

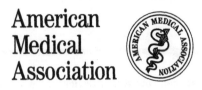

Guide to
Talking to
Your Doctor

Angela Perry, MD

Medical Editor

JOHN WILEY & SONS, INC.

New York • Chichester • Weinheim • Brisbane • Singapore • Toronto

Published by John Wiley & Sons, Inc.
Published simultaneously in Canada

Design and production by Navta Associates, Inc.

This publication is designed to provide accurate and authoritative information in regard to the subject matter covered. It is sold with the understanding that the publisher is not engaged in rendering professional services. If professional advice or other expert assistance is required, the services of a competent professional person should be sought.

The recommendations and information in this book are appropriate in most cases; however, they are not a substitute for a medical diagnosis. For specific information concerning a medical condition, the AMA suggests that you consult a physician. The names of organizations, products, or alternative therapies appearing in this book are given for informational purposes only. Their inclusion does not imply AMA endorsement, nor does the omission of any organization, product, or alternative therapy indicate AMA disapproval.

Photo credits: p. 4, © AMA; p. 12, © PhotoDisc; p. 36, © Corbis; p. 66, © Stone/Bruce Ayres; p. 80, © PhotoDisc; p. 110, © PhotoDisc.

Library of Congress Cataloging-in-Publication Data:

The American Medical Association guide to talking to your doctor / American Medical Association.
    p. ; cm
  Includes index.
  ISBN 0-471-41410-7 (paper)
  1. Physician and patient. 2. Interpersonal communication. 3. Patient participation. I. Title: Guide to talking to your doctor. II. American Medical Association.
  [DNLM: 1. Physician-Patient Relations—Popular Works. 2. Communication—Popular Works. 3. Patient Participation—Popular Works. W 62 A5115 2001]
  RA727.3 .A53 2001
  610.69'6—dc21   2001024711

10 9 8 7 6 5 4 3 2 1

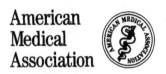

American
Medical
Association

Foreword

Most of us think of medicine as a high-tech science, which it is. But for doctors, the core of their practice is their interaction with patients. Good medicine is a partnership between doctor and patient, whether the doctor is performing a physical examination or listening carefully to a patient's description of his or her symptoms. The *American Medical Association Guide to Talking to Your Doctor* is designed to help nurture and strengthen this relationship.

If you are reading this book, you have decided to take responsibility for your health and you want to learn how to get the information you need to help you make informed decisions about your healthcare. You may have older or younger family members whom you accompany to the doctor, and you want to help them get the best care possible. Perhaps you need a specialist or have moved to another town; this book explains the resources you can tap into to find a doctor in your new community. One of these resources is the American Medical Association Web site at http://www.ama-assn.org (click on Doctor Finder).

This book gives you information about how to prepare for a doctor's visit or phone call. Should you tell your doctor about an alternative treatment you are using? Should you ask about a medication you saw advertised on television? If you need to undergo a diagnostic test, how do you find out how the test is done and what to expect during the test? At some time in our lives, each of us will have a health problem that we would rather not discuss. The section in the book on talking about sensitive subjects gives you some helpful tips on how to bring the subject up and gives you the encouragement to do so.

We at the American Medical Association hope that this information will help you feel more confident and comfortable the next time you visit your doctor. We wish you and your family good health.

American Medical Association

The American Medical Association

Robert A. Musacchio   *Senior Vice President, Business and Membership*

Anthony J. Frankos   *Vice President, Business Products*

AMA Press

Mary Lou S. White   *Editorial Director*

Patricia Dragisic   *Senior Managing Editor*

Donna Kotulak   *Managing Editor*

Robin Fitzpatrick Husayko   *Senior Editor*

Claudia Appeldorn   *Copy Editor*

Mary Ann Albanese   *Image Coordinator*

Reuben Rios   *Editorial Assistant*

Roger Banther   *Editorial Assistant*

Medical Editor

Angela Perry, MD

Writers

Steven Michaels

Ellen Hughes

Acknowledgments

Bruce Blehart, JD   *Health/Law Litigation*

Arthur Elster, MD   *Integrated Clinical and Public Health/Science*

Linda Emanuel, MD   *Ethical Standards*

Kathryn Meshenberg   *Ethical Standards*

Leatha Tiggelaar   *Science, Technology, and Public Health*

Patricia Watson   *Ethical Standards*

Mathew Wynia, MD, MPH   *Ethical Standards*

Contents

Introduction

Today the emphasis in health and medical care is on prevention. The *American Medical Association Guide to Talking to Your
Doctor* focuses on the importance of an effective patient-doctor
relationship in improving and maintaining your health and
reducing your health risks. Use this book as a tool to become an
informed, active healthcare participant and to take control of
your health and medical care.

In many patient-doctor relationships, the doctor is the more
active participant. The doctor talks and the patient listens, the
doctor asks questions and the patient provides answers. This
limited communication can cause problems for both doctor and
patient and can have a negative impact on the patient's health
and medical care. For example, if you don't understand the
information your doctor provides, you may become confused
and frustrated and lose confidence in the doctor. You may even
stop following his or her instructions, and, as a result, your
treatment may not be effective and your health problems could
get worse.

Many people are hesitant to talk to their doctor even though
they want to ask questions or discuss their health problems.

Embarrassment and fear of bad news are two common reasons for not talking to the doctor. Other possible explanations include both real and imagined time limitations, reluctance to question the doctor's authority, limited ability to speak English, feeling that one's questions and concerns are unimportant, and not wanting to appear stupid. But to get all you need from your medical care and make informed health-related choices, you need to assume an active role in your own health and medical care. Your doctor relies on information only you can provide, such as details about symptoms, before he or she can make an accurate diagnosis or provide proper treatment. He or she also must have confidence in your ability to follow instructions carefully so that your treatment can be effective.

Your doctor should encourage and support your active participation and always should be willing to take time to address your questions and concerns. The highest levels of satisfaction with medical care and the best treatment outcomes occur when both doctor and patient communicate openly and honestly and work together closely to achieve shared goals.

To become an active partner you need to listen carefully, ask questions, discuss treatment options and goals, participate in decision-making, follow instructions carefully, know what to expect from your treatment, and provide feedback. All of this requires clear communication between you and your doctor. Although it may be difficult at first, you will discover that you and your doctor will gradually work together more easily as you get to know each other. Both you and your doctor will benefit.

The book is divided into six chapters. "Choosing a Doctor" helps you find what you are looking for in a physician and tells you how to go about the search. Use the checklists and record-keeping forms in the second chapter, "What Your Doctor Wants to Know about You," to keep your and family members' health histories. "Talking about Your Health and Medical

Care," "Talking for Others," and "Talking about Sensitive Subjects" give you guidelines for discussing your health risks and healthcare needs with your doctor. These chapters also prepare you for talking to doctors for members of your family, such as a child or an older parent, and encourage you to overcome any embarrassment or hesitation you may have about talking openly and honestly with your doctor about sensitive subjects such as sex. The "Special Situations" chapter helps you evaluate the benefits and risks of treatment options such as surgery that you may be faced with and enables you to make an informed decision about an appropriate treatment for you.

At the end of the book, the resources section and the glossary help you find information about specific topics and understand terms you may have heard or read or that your doctor may use in your visits. The resources section gives the names, addresses (including some e-mail addresses), phone numbers (usually toll-free), and Web sites of diverse associations and organizations that provide information on health or healthcare-related topics. The resources section is subdivided into segments such as advocacy, clinical trials, diseases and conditions, health information Web sites, home-care services and hospice, long-term care and housing, mental health, rehabilitation, and self-help and support.

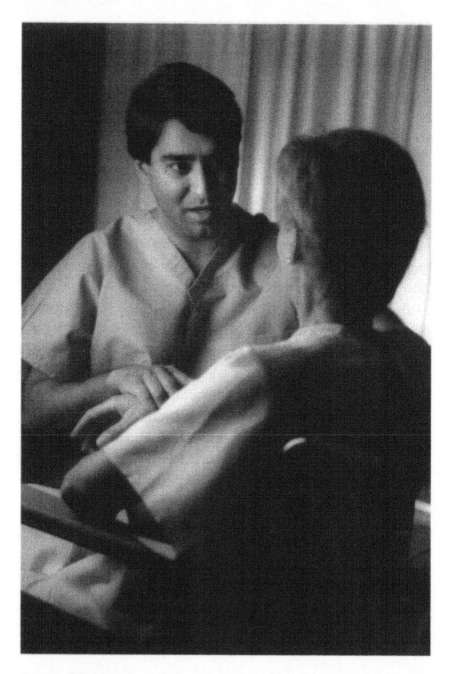

An Active Partnership

Your relationship with your doctor is a working partnership with a common goal: to keep you healthy. When choosing a doctor, look for someone who takes the time to listen to your concerns and who answers your questions clearly and in a reassuring tone. You want to have confidence in the doctor and feel comfortable enough with him or her to be able to express your concerns openly. The more open and honest you are with your doctor, the better able he or she will be to evaluate your health risks, diagnose an illness, and provide effective treatment.

1

Choosing a Doctor

There are many reasons why you might need to choose a doctor. A change in health insurance, a move to another city, the need for a specialist, your doctor's retirement, or a communication problem with your present physician all could be factors. If you or a family member recently had a baby, you need a pediatrician or a family practitioner to care for the child. Take your time and ask questions while you are in the process of choosing the physician who is right for you. Don't make this important decision in a rush. And don't wait until you are really sick or you have a medical emergency to explore your options.

What Are You Looking For?

Whether you are looking for a primary care physician or a specialist, consider your own preferences and needs. You can easily find a great deal of information about a doctor—from board certification (see page 49) and education to practice philosophy and number of years in practice. What is important to you? Perhaps you prefer a physician who is older than you are, or of the same sex. Would you like your doctor's cultural background to be similar to yours? Are you more drawn to a person who is warm and personally connected to you, or are you more interested in a doctor's technical knowledge? If a doctor's technical knowledge is more important to you, look for a doctor who has a teaching position at a university or has clinical privileges at a respected hospital.

Choosing a Doctor

Q I'm interested in finding a new doctor in my community. What kind of information on physicians can I get using one of those telephone or online doctor-finder services?

A Most doctor-selection services organize physicians by medical practice and location. Some provide information about their background, interests, education, and training. Expanded listings may include photographs of the physicians and their professional achievements. Patients can have a number of different reasons for choosing a physician. For example, some may prefer a doctor who speaks their native language. Or they may feel more comfortable with a physician of the same sex or about the same age.

Other Issues to Consider

Besides personal preference and philosophy, you also will have to consider issues of time, location, and cost. A doctor's office hours or location may enter into your decision. Find out if you will have to make an appointment far in advance and if his or her office hours and days are convenient for you. Who can see you when your doctor is away or otherwise unavailable? How far will you have to travel to an appointment?

If you are in a managed care plan, your choices are narrowed because you need to choose your doctor from a list of those in the plan. Or you may need a doctor who will accept Medicare. If you do not have health coverage through work, or if you have an individual health plan with limited benefits or no insurance at all, you will have to consider cost along with all the other factors.

Under many health insurance plans, changing doctors means selecting another from the list of physicians whose services are included in your plan's coverage. Before you make a choice, ask around. Other people in the same plan may be able to recommend a physician whose approach would be good for you.

Should You Change Doctors?

Q I have been seeing the same doctor for 10 years and suddenly I am having a hard time making an appointment. When I do get an appointment, I have to wait at least an hour before seeing her. I don't know what to do because I have always had confidence in this doctor and I respect her medical knowledge. Should I complain to her or someone in her office or should I just get another doctor?

A Because you like and respect your doctor, you should see if there is a way to solve the problem before you look for another doctor. It's important that you have confidence in your doctor. In a calm, courteous way, let the doctor know about the difficulty you've been having getting in to see her. She is probably unaware of the problem and will be happy to have your input. If the problem persists or gets worse and you feel no effort has been made to improve it, then you might consider finding another doctor.

How to Go about Choosing a Doctor

You can choose a doctor in a number of ways. Ask friends and relatives about their doctors and if they have had good experiences. Ask specifically why they like their doctor; you might not have the same preferences. You also can ask medical specialists and other healthcare professionals for recommendations. Check with a nearby hospital or medical school. An old standby is to ask a doctor the name of his or her doctor; this usually works well when you need a specialist ("Who checks your eyes?" for example). Local medical societies can give you the names of doctors who are accepting new patients in your area. And many hospitals offer physician-referral services at no charge.

The newest way to find a doctor is through an online doctor-referral service (see "General Health Information" Web sites starting on page 171). These services will be able to provide you with most, if not all, of the above-mentioned criteria. Whether you need to stick to a list of physicians or are free to choose for yourself, you can find out more about any physician by searching Doctor Finder on the American Medical Association's Web site. Access it from the AMA's home page at http://www.ama-assn.org (see page 173). Here you can locate doctors in your area by specialty and find out specifics about their medical training, specialty certification, and practice. After you have made your decision, have a copy of your medical records sent to your new doctor.

Your Rights and Responsibilities as a Healthcare Consumer

People who communicate openly and effectively with their physician and other healthcare professionals and who also know their rights as healthcare consumers are better equipped to make informed decisions about their health and healthcare. You have the following rights as a healthcare consumer:

- To receive considerate and respectful care without regard to your sex, age, race, ethnic background, religion, or income.

- To be fully informed, in terms you can understand, about your disease or condition, potential treatment options, and possible outcomes.

- To know the names and roles of the people who are providing your treatment (such as doctors, nurses, therapists, and other healthcare professionals).

- To participate in decisions about your healthcare and to consent to or refuse a given course of treatment. If you refuse treatment, you are entitled to consider other available, realistic, and medically appropriate treatment options.

- To seek second opinions.

- To change doctors if you are not satisfied with the care you are receiving.

- To put in place advance directives such as a living will or durable power of attorney for healthcare to help ensure that your healthcare preferences are honored if you are not able to speak for yourself.

- To have your privacy respected regarding all aspects of your health and healthcare.

- To have your medical records kept confidential, except in cases where reporting is allowed or required by law (such as for review by insurers or for public health concerns). Confidentiality is emphasized in these circumstances. Your written permission is required to release your medical records to other interested parties.

- To review your medical records and have the information explained and interpreted for you, unless restricted by law in your state.

- To receive reasonable responses to reasonable requests for service.

- To receive reasonable continuity of care.

- To be able to refuse to participate in research studies. A person considering whether to participate in research studies is entitled to be fully informed about such studies before giving consent.

- To receive and review a bill for services provided, and to have that bill explained to you.

You also have responsibilities as a healthcare consumer. By becoming actively involved in your healthcare, you will be able to make informed choices that will help you to improve and maintain your health for the rest of your life. To be a responsible, informed healthcare consumer, you should do the following:

- Provide complete and accurate information to healthcare professionals about your health history, including past illnesses, hospitalizations, and use of medication.

- Become involved in healthcare decisions.

- Ask questions whenever you do not understand any information or instructions from your doctor or other healthcare professional.
- Communicate openly and honestly with your doctor about your health and healthcare.
- Work closely with your doctor.
- Follow your doctor's instructions completely and carefully.
- Tell your doctor if you have problems with your treatment.
- Acknowledge the effect that your lifestyle can have on your health and take responsibility for improving your lifestyle.
- Become familiar with the benefits provided by your healthcare plan.

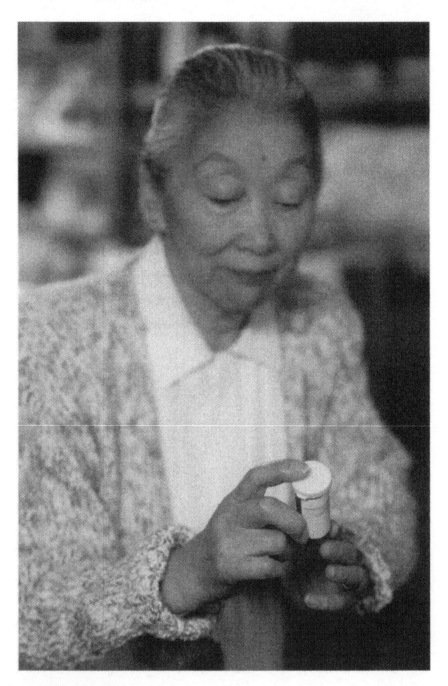

Providing Information

To help your doctor make an accurate diagnosis of a medical condition or recommend effective treatment, you need to give him or her accurate information, including details about any medications you are taking. It's a good idea to bring all your medications in their containers with you to the doctor's office so he or she can evaluate them. Information about your medications is especially helpful if your doctor is considering prescribing another medication for you.

2

What Your Doctor Wants to Know about You

Your doctor needs certain information about you, such as details about your past and current health, your previous medical care, and your health habits, behaviors, and attitudes. This information will help your doctor get to know you better so that he or she can provide the best possible care. This information is also the foundation upon which you and your doctor will base your relationship.

Regular checkups and screening tests are essential for continuity of care. In the past, most people had a yearly physical examination and underwent a standard series of screening tests. Because each person is different, with different health needs, this is no longer considered a practical approach to medical care; seeing every person at the same intervals and giving every person the same tests are not logical, practical, or affordable. Therefore your doctor will base your checkups, tests, and treatments on factors that are specific to you, such as your gender, age, personal health history, family health history, and lifestyle.

Personal Health History

Your doctor keeps a record of your health and medical care at the office. The information collected in these medical files is what makes up your personal health history. The files are updated each time you visit your doctor.

It is a good idea to keep track of your own health history. Knowledge of your personal health history can help you understand your health risks and get the medical care you need. Your health history should include essential information about your health and your lifestyle. The information can be broken down into several main categories, such as personal information, medical history, social history, and preventive health history.

The following checklist will help you complete your health history. Although the list includes a wide variety of diseases and conditions, it is merely a guide and is not meant to be comprehensive. Use the list to jog your memory; be sure to include all diseases and conditions you have had, even if you do not find them on this checklist.

GENERAL

   ☐ Underweight   ☐ Obesity
   ☐ Overweight   ☐ Eating disorder

SKIN

   ☐ Acne   ☐ Skin cancer
   ☐ Eczema   ☐ Skin changes
   ☐ Rash   ☐ Other_____

HEAD (INCLUDING EYES, EARS, AND NOSE)

- ☐ Seasonal allergies
- ☐ Farsightedness
- ☐ Nearsightedness
- ☐ Cataracts
- ☐ Glaucoma
- ☐ Headaches (tension headaches, migraines)
- ☐ Hearing problems
- ☐ Otitis media (ear infections)
- ☐ Tinnitus (ringing in the ears)
- ☐ Nosebleeds
- ☐ Sinusitis (sinus infections)

THROAT AND NECK

- ☐ Enlarged glands
- ☐ Goiter
- ☐ Thyroid disorders
- ☐ Hoarseness

ENDOCRINE SYSTEM

- ☐ Diabetes
- ☐ Thyroid disorders

BONES, MUSCLES, AND JOINTS

- ☐ Arthritis
- ☐ Back pain
- ☐ Bunions
- ☐ Gout
- ☐ Joint weakness
- ☐ Muscle weakness
- ☐ Peripheral vascular disease (pain in calves when walking)
- ☐ Other_____

BLOOD

- ☐ Anemia
- ☐ Coagulation problems
- ☐ Phlebitis
- ☐ Thalassemia

BRAIN

- ☐ Epilepsy or seizures
- ☐ Paralysis

HEART AND CIRCULATION

- ☐ Angina (chest pain)
- ☐ Edema (swelling, especially the ankles)
- ☐ Heart attack
- ☐ Heart failure
- ☐ Heart murmur
- ☐ Heart rhythm disorders
- ☐ High blood pressure
- ☐ Stroke
- ☐ Varicose veins

RESPIRATORY TRACT

- ☐ Asthma
- ☐ Bronchitis
- ☐ Colds
- ☐ Cough (chronic)
- ☐ Emphysema
- ☐ Pleurisy
- ☐ Pneumonia
- ☐ Shortness of breath

DIGESTIVE TRACT

- ☐ Bloody stools
- ☐ Changes in bowel habits
- ☐ Cirrhosis
- ☐ Constipation
- ☐ Diarrhea
- ☐ Hemorrhoids
- ☐ Hepatitis
- ☐ Hernia
- ☐ Gallbladder disease
- ☐ Gallstones
- ☐ Gas (chronic)
- ☐ Gastritis
- ☐ Gastroesophageal reflux
- ☐ Incontinence
- ☐ Irritable bowel syndrome
- ☐ Pancreatitis
- ☐ Spastic colon
- ☐ Ulcer
- ☐ Other_____

URINARY TRACT

- ☐ Bladder disorders
- ☐ Blood in the urine
- ☐ Frequent urination
- ☐ Incontinence
- ☐ Kidney disease
- ☐ Kidney stones
- ☐ Prostate disease
- ☐ Other_____

WOMEN'S HEALTH

- ☐ Breast lumps (benign)
- ☐ Breast cancer
- ☐ Ovarian cysts
- ☐ Uterine fibroids
- ☐ Painful periods
- ☐ Irregular periods
- ☐ Premenstrual syndrome (PMS)
- ☐ Other_____

MENTAL HEALTH

- ☐ Anxiety
- ☐ Depression
- ☐ Seasonal affective disorder (SAD)
- ☐ Other_____

CANCER

- ☐ Bladder
- ☐ Blood (leukemia)
- ☐ Bone
- ☐ Brain
- ☐ Breast
- ☐ Colon
- ☐ Liver
- ☐ Lung
- ☐ Lymph system (lymphoma)
- ☐ Mouth
- ☐ Ovary
- ☐ Pancreas
- ☐ Prostate
- ☐ Rectum
- ☐ Skin
- ☐ Stomach
- ☐ Uterus
- ☐ Other_____

Encourage your spouse or partner to keep a personal health history of his or her own. Your medical records are updated each time you receive treatment. The contents of your health history are kept confidential. Keep your own copy of your health history and update it as needed. Although you may be tempted to rely on your memory (or the memories of others), dates and specific details related to your health and medical care are easy to forget.

YOUR PERSONAL HEALTH HISTORY

Personal Information

Full name _____

Gender ☐ Male ☐ Female

Birth date _____ Age _____

Birthplace _____

Racial or ethnic background _____

Medical History

Current diseases, conditions, or injuries _____

_____

Previous diseases, conditions, or injuries, including those during
    childhood _____

_____

Previous treatments or procedures (such as surgery), including
    those during childhood _____

_____

Blood transfusion (dates)_____

Mental illness _____

Current prescription medications _____

_____

Current nonprescription medications, including vitamins or other
    supplements _____

Drug allergies or reactions _____

Eye exams (dates)_____

Ear exams (dates) _____

Dental visits (dates) _____

(continued)

Gynecological History (women only)

Age at menstruation _____

Date of last period _____

Age at menopause _____

Hormone replacement therapy (for how long?) _____

Abnormal Pap smears _____

Date of most recent Pap smear _____

Abnormal mammograms _____

Date of most recent mammogram _____

Gynecological procedures and operations (dates) _____

Reproductive History (women only)

Number of pregnancies (dates) _____

Number of live births (dates) _____

Number of miscarriages (dates) _____

Number of abortions (dates) _____

Birth control methods _____

Urological History (men only)

Prostate problems _____

Urination problems _____

Sexual dysfunction (such as erectile dysfunction) _____

Urinary tract surgery (dates) _____

Social History (personal information)

Marital status _____

Number of children _____

Sexual activity _____

(continued)

Preventive Health History (lifestyle factors)

Tobacco use _____

Alcohol use _____

Other drug use _____

Exercise (regularity, type, amount) _____

Diet _____

Methods for coping with day-to-day stress _____

Seat belt use _____

Practicing safer sex (such as using condoms if not in a monogamous
   relationship) _____

Use of safety equipment (such as bicycle helmets and knee pads)

_____

Smoke alarms and carbon monoxide detectors in home _____

Gun ownership _____

Immunizations—diphtheria, tetanus, and pertussis; *Haemophilus
   influenzae* type b; polio; pneumococcal disease; influenza; measles,
   mumps, and rubella; hepatitis A and B (dates)_____

Alternative or complementary healthcare practices _____

Doctors

Current primary care physician (name, address, phone number)

_____

Previous primary care physicians (names, addresses, phone numbers)

_____

_____

Specialists (names, addresses, phone numbers) _____

_____

Health Insurance

Health insurance company and group policy number _____

Your ID number _____

Health insurance company's phone number _____

Filling Out Medical Forms

Q I am a man who has had problems performing sexually for some time. I don't think it's anybody else's business. I'm getting older, and I've accepted it. Recently I had to fill out a medical history form at my doctor's office that asked questions about my sex life. Needless to say, I didn't answer these questions. What reason could there be for asking such questions?

A Your doctor is not just being nosy. Yes, sexual function may slow somewhat as we age, but it shouldn't stop altogether. There are legitimate medical reasons for asking these questions, and your doctor may be able to help you. For example, you may have an underlying health condition that is affecting your ability to perform sexually. High blood pressure, heart disease, or diabetes can cause erectile dysfunction (formerly known as impotence). Drinking an excessive amount of alcohol can affect your ability to have and maintain an erection. Or perhaps a medication you are taking, such as a tranquilizer, is the cause and needs to be adjusted. You should always be honest when filling out health history forms. Let your doctor make the diagnosis. Effective treatments are available for most sexual problems.

Confidentiality of Medical Records

Your medical records contain personal information about your health and medical care. Protecting the privacy of medical records has become a much-debated issue involving consumer rights, healthcare policy, and medical ethics. There are currently no uniform national laws or regulations to protect the privacy and confidentiality of patients' medical information, and state laws and regulations in this area vary from state to state.

Protecting confidentiality of medical records is an important aspect of the patient-doctor relationship. Most people believe that this information should be viewed and used only by their doctor and authorized office staff. Their fear is that a third party might gain access to their medical records without their consent. People who could have access to medical records might include the following:

- Health insurance plan administrators
- Health insurance plan claims processors
- Hospital staff with access to the hospital's information system
- Human resources staff at your workplace
- Pharmacists (to check prescription drug records)
- Companies that collect healthcare information about people who apply for health or life insurance
- Anyone with access to healthcare, public health, and statistical databases

Although the information in your medical records is about your health and medical care, the records are not your property. According to law, a person's medical records are the property of the healthcare provider who produced them, such as a doctor or a hospital. Your right to look at your records, correct errors, and control access to and disclosure of the information they contain without your consent is limited. You are, however, entitled to look at your medical records and to have a copy of them. If you want to see or if you need a copy of your medical records, ask your doctor or healthcare provider.

Your Child's Health History

In addition to keeping track of your own health history, it is a good idea to keep health histories for your children. Fill in the requested information, and update it as needed. To avoid confusion, be sure to fill out a separate form for each child. Pass these health histories (or copies) along to your children when they're adults so that they can use this valuable information to complete their personal health histories.

Privacy in the Pediatrician's Office

Q My son is 13 years old. I have had a good relationship with his pediatrician since my son was born, but the doctor recently retired and a younger doctor has taken his place. I don't especially like this new doctor's attitude. She talks to my son more than she talks to me, and she always wants to examine my son alone. I don't think my son is old enough to speak for himself.

A Your son's new pediatrician is following standard procedure by talking to your son in private. She can ask him about sensitive health-related topics such as drug use or sexual activity that he might not answer truthfully or in full when you are present. You want the best possible healthcare for your son, and having your son and his doctor talk alone is one way for him to get it. Keep in mind that she is your son's doctor, not yours. If your son has a good rapport with his doctor, and the healthcare and the medical advice she is giving seem sound, it might be wise to step back and let the relationship continue.

Schedule of Childhood Immunizations

Here is the recommended schedule of immunizations for most children, which may change as a result of medical research and as new vaccines are developed. Your child's doctor will follow the most current schedule and can recommend the best timing for each vaccination. Be sure to tell the doctor if your child has ever had seizures or if he or she is ill at the scheduled time of immunization.

AGE	VACCINE
Birth–2 months	Hepatitis B
1–4 months	Hepatitis B
2 months	DTaP, Hib, IPV, PCV
4 months	DTaP, Hib, IPV, PCV
6 months	DTaP, Hib, PCV
6–18 months	Hepatitis B, IPV
12–15 months	Hib, MMR, PCV
15–18 months	DTaP
24 months–18 years	Hepatitis A (in selected regions)
4–6 years	DTaP, IPV, MMR
11–12 years	MMR (if not given previously), hepatitis B (if not given previously), Td (if at least 5 years have elapsed since the last dose of DTaP)
11–16 years	DTaP

KEY

DTaP	Diphtheria and tetanus toxoids and acellular pertussis
Hib	*Haemophilus influenzae* type b
IPV	Inactivated poliovirus
MMR	Measles, mumps, rubella
PCV	Pneumococcal conjugate vaccine
Td	Tetanus and diphtheria toxoids

YOUR CHILD'S HEALTH HISTORY

Personal Information

Full name _____

Gender   ☐ Male   ☐ Female

Birth date _____ Age _____

Birthplace _____

Racial or ethnic background _____

Medical History

Current diseases, conditions, or injuries _____

_____

Previous diseases, conditions, or injuries _____

_____

Previous treatments or procedures (such as surgery) _____

_____

Mental illness _____

Current prescription medications _____

_____

Current nonprescription medications, including vitamins _____

_____

Drug allergies or reactions _____

Eye exams (dates) _____

Ear exams (dates) _____

Dental visits (dates) _____

Social History

Parents' marital status _____

Number of siblings _____

(continued)

Year in school _____

Adopted _____

Preventive Health History (lifestyle factors)

Exercise (regularity, type, amount) _____

Diet _____

Seat belt use _____

Use of safety equipment (such as bicycle helmets and knee pads)

_____

Immunizations (see chart) _____

Doctors

Current primary care physician (name, address, phone number)

_____

_____

Previous primary care physicians (names, addresses, phone numbers)

_____

_____

Specialists (names, addresses, phone numbers) _____

_____

Health Insurance

Health insurance company and group policy number _____

_____

Your child's ID number _____

Health insurance company's phone number _____

Family Health History

Although you may not be aware of it, your family health history has a significant impact on your health and is an important supplement to your personal health history. The health histories of your grandparents, parents, aunts, uncles, siblings, and children include information that may reflect on your health and the health of other family members. The reason that some diseases have a tendency to run in families is often a matter of biology or the genes we inherit from our parents (half from our father and half from our mother). Genes are the basic units of biological information that determine many of our characteristics, including a predisposition to developing certain diseases or conditions.

Some of the diseases that are linked to both genes and environmental factors such as lifestyle (including diabetes and heart disease) are common, while others (such as cystic fibrosis and sickle cell disease), which are linked to a single defective gene, are less common. Many of these diseases are life-threatening. Specific health information about your blood relatives can help your doctor anticipate, prevent, or treat these diseases. A family health history also can be useful to help predict and protect the health of your children, grandchildren, and later generations in your family.

Do not assume because a certain disease or condition seems to run in your family that you or a family member will necessarily develop it. Even more significant in the development of health problems that tend to run in families are factors other than genes, such as environment or lifestyle, which usually can be modified. Also, prevalence of the disease or condition in your family and the closeness of your blood relationship to relatives who have or have had it are important factors in your chances of developing that disease or condition.

Your family health history is an invaluable tool that you and your doctor can use to determine your and your children's health risks and the steps you and your children can take to stay healthy. Making note of family behaviors and health habits also will prove valuable in evaluating your health risks. Once you have gathered and organized this vital information, you will be better prepared to take control of your health and medical care. You also will be more likely to work with your doctor to make lifestyle changes and to schedule any needed screening tests.

A family health history resembles a family tree except that it contains medical information rather than historical information about your ancestors. To create a complete family health history, you will need to include specific, detailed, health-related information about the following people:

- Father
- Mother
- Sisters
- Brothers
- Grandparents (paternal and maternal)
- Uncles (paternal and maternal)
- Aunts (paternal and maternal)
- You
- Your spouse or partner
- Your children

Be as thorough as possible, and provide the following information about each person:

- Full name
- Birth date
- Age at death
- Cause of death
- Major diseases and conditions

- Age of onset of diseases and conditions
- Specific symptoms of specific diseases and conditions
- Whether the relative is from your father's or your mother's side of the family

Pay special attention to the occurrence of any of the following common chronic diseases and conditions; they tend to run in families.

- Alcoholism or other drug addiction
- Allergies, including reactions to medications
- Alzheimer's disease
- Arthritis
- Cancer (type? age at diagnosis?)
- Depression or other mood disorders
- Diabetes
- Heart disease
- High blood pressure
- Kidney disease
- Schizophrenia

To complete your family health history, include information about:

- Multiple births
- Miscarriages, stillbirths, infant deaths
- Deaths from disease in children and young adults

Medications

Many people take one or more medications every day. These medications may have been prescribed by a doctor or purchased over-the-counter. Your doctor needs information about all of the prescription and nonprescription medications that you are currently taking. Your doctor also will need to know how much alcohol you drink and whether you use any illegal drugs. All of this information is important because any of these substances can interact with the medications your doctor prescribes, potentially altering their effectiveness and safety.

Make a list of all of the medications (including over-the-counter medications) you are taking, including dosages (the amount and how often you take the medication each day). If you are seeing more than one doctor, be sure to list all of the medications from all of the doctors you are seeing. Bring the list along whenever you visit your doctor. He or she needs this information to evaluate the appropriateness and success of your ongoing drug treatment. If you are taking several prescription medications, your doctor may prefer that you bring in the actual medications rather than a list. For older people, the doctor may ask the patient to bring in all medications so they can discuss each one. This will help eliminate any errors or confusion and will give your doctor the opportunity to make sure that your prescriptions are correct and safe to take together.

To check the accuracy of your prescriptions, your doctor needs to know the following:

- Name of the medication
- Why you are taking it
- How much you are taking (dose)
- How often you take the medication
- When you take it (time of day)

Costly Medication

Q The medication my doctor has prescribed is very expensive, and my insurance does not cover the cost of medications. I don't think I can afford it. What should I do?

A Tell your doctor about your concerns. He or she may be able to substitute a generic form of the drug or a similar, less costly drug. It also may be possible for your doctor to give you free samples of the medication or help you enroll in a patient assistance program sponsored by a pharmaceutical company. In some cases, a doctor may recommend participating in a clinical trial that is studying a particular medication to treat a condition.

Self-treatment

Today many people use a wide variety of over-the-counter medications to treat a number of conditions, from colds and flu to arthritis. Along with information about the prescription medications you are taking, your list should include the same type of information about any over-the-counter medications you are taking, such as:

- Pain and fever relievers, including aspirin, acetaminophen, ibuprofen, ketoprofen, and naproxen
- Diet aids
- Sleeping pills
- Cough syrups
- Cold medications
- Allergy relievers, including nasal sprays
- Antacids and other ulcer medications
- Vitamins and minerals
- Melatonin or other nutritional supplements
- Herbal remedies
- Homeopathic remedies
- Laxatives
- Eye drops

Before he or she can properly prescribe medication, your doctor also needs to know the following:

- If you have any drug allergies
- If you have ever had an unpleasant or unexpected reaction to any medication
- If you are (or could be) pregnant
- If you are breast-feeding
- If you have problems swallowing pills

Many drug companies advertise their new prescription medications directly to healthcare consumers. You have probably seen ads for a variety of drugs on television, in magazines and newspapers, and elsewhere. Some of these medications may be used to treat a condition that you or a loved one have. If you have questions about any of these drugs, talk to your doctor. While the ads may be persuasive, remember that your doctor is always your most reliable source of information about any medication. Some medications may interfere with the effects of other medications you are already taking, possibly causing side effects, or they may not be safe for people with your medical history.

If you have any questions or concerns about your medication or treatment plan, or if you need more information, do not hesitate to ask your doctor. Getting the help and advice you need when you need it is vital for the success of your treatment plan. For additional information, see page 50.

Telling Your Doctor about Alternative Treatments

Q Should I tell my doctor that I plan to take the herbal supplement ginkgo biloba? I'm 75 and my sister-in-law, who is the same age, says her memory has improved after taking ginkgo biloba for 2 years. I would like to try it but I know that many doctors disapprove of alternative therapies. I am taking the prescription medications warfarin, a blood thinner, and lovastatin, a cholesterol-lowering drug. It can't hurt me to take ginkgo biloba, too, can it?

A Most medications, whether available by prescription or over-the-counter, can interact with other medications, so it is vital to be honest and direct with your doctor about what you are taking—or what you are thinking about taking. Bleeding problems can occur when you take ginkgo biloba with the blood thinner warfarin. For the same reason, you should not take aspirin if you are taking ginkgo biloba or warfarin. Like warfarin, aspirin has blood-thinning properties.

Lifestyle

The lifestyle choices you make today will have a strong impact on your health in the future. Making the right choices now can help keep you healthy, while making the wrong choices can put your health at risk and even threaten your life. A number of diseases and conditions can be traced directly to risky behavior throughout a person's lifetime. These behaviors include eating a poor diet, exercising too little, smoking, abusing alcohol or other drugs, or having unsafe sex. Avoiding risky behaviors and living a healthier lifestyle are easy ways to prevent many diseases, injuries, and disabilities.

To provide the best possible medical care, your doctor will need to know about your lifestyle. Be open and honest with your doctor. Do not hold back any information, even very personal information that would seem embarrassing in a social situation. Your doctor is likely to ask you about the following:

- Your eating habits
- Your sleep habits
- Your exercise habits
- Whether you smoke cigarettes or cigars, chew tobacco, or drink alcohol
- Whether you use or have ever used illegal drugs
- Your sexual habits (such as whether you have more than one sexual partner)
- Other aspects of your daily routine (such as your driving habits and how you deal with day-to-day stress)

Healthy Habits

Q My friend's doctor told her that by losing as little as 10 pounds and exercising more she could probably get her blood pressure down to a healthier level without the need for medication. I'm already taking medication for high blood pressure. Should I ask my doctor if losing weight and exercising more might make it possible for me to stop taking the medication?

A It's always a good idea to ask your doctor about lifestyle changes that can improve your health. Your doctor will probably encourage you to try to exercise more and lose weight and come in for regular checkups to monitor your blood pressure and see if it has improved. In addition to lowering your blood pressure, exercise and weight loss give you many other health benefits, including a lower risk of heart disease, type 2 diabetes, and some kinds of cancer.

Your doctor also wants to know about your long-term health-related goals. For example, do you intend to become pregnant? Are you trying to quit smoking? Are you trying to lose weight? Your doctor is also interested in knowing your attitudes about health and medical care. Be sure to tell your doctor about any alternative therapies you are using or have used in the past, such as chiropractic, acupuncture, or homeopathy. People often are reluctant to talk to their physicians about alternative treatments for fear of disapproval, but your doctor needs to know about all treatments you are using, including alternative treatments, so he or she can provide the best possible healthcare.

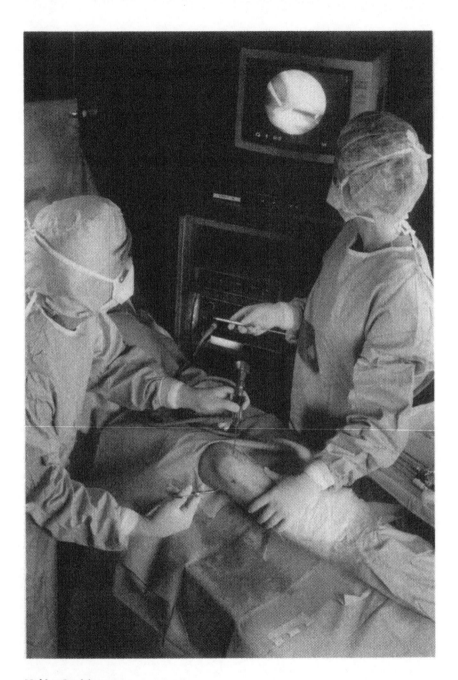

Making Decisions

When faced with having surgery, don't hesitate to ask your doctor questions about the procedure, including why he or she recommends it, what you can expect, what the procedure involves, and what the nonsurgical alternatives are, if any. Ask about the potential benefits and risks of having the surgery, and make sure that the benefits outweigh the risks. Always keep in mind that being an active participant in your healthcare helps you make informed decisions.

3

Talking about Your Health and Medical Care

The following sections will show you how being prepared will help you get the advice and information you need while making the best use of your time and your doctor's time. As you will see, a little planning goes a long way.

Planning in Advance
What to Say to the Doctor

Your doctor probably receives many more phone calls each day than he or she could possibly handle. When you call, it is unlikely that you will be able to speak directly to your doctor. A patient's calls are routinely screened by trained staff (such as a receptionist, nurse, or nurse practitioner) who determine the nature of the problem and decide whether a patient needs to see or speak with the doctor or if the call can be handled in some other way. Often the patient must leave a detailed message with a nurse or a receptionist and wait for the doctor to return the call.

To avoid potential problems, it is a good idea to take time to get organized before you call your doctor's office. Some simple preparation will help you to make the most efficient use of your doctor's time and ensure that you get the information you need. Write down the most important points you want to cover in your call—including the reason you are calling, a description of your symptoms, and the questions you want to ask.

Mental Health Benefits

The Mental Health Parity Act of 1996 requires most employers to offer mental health benefits, just as they offer medical and surgical benefits. Businesses with fewer than 50 employees are exempt; the law might allow other businesses to be exempt based on cost increases. The final rules of the Department of Health and Human Services that took effect in 1998 require group plans to provide the same monetary limits for mental health benefits that they do for medical benefits. You should be notified by your employer if your plan is exempt from these rules. Because of a sunset provision (which requires periodic review for worthiness), the Mental Health Parity Act might not apply to benefits after September 30, 2001.

Before you seek treatment by a mental health professional, check if your health insurance plan provides coverage for mental illness. If you are covered, it is important that you understand the mental health benefits provided in your plan. Here are some issues to consider:

- Does your insurance plan include mental health benefits?
- Is preapproval necessary?
- Do you need a referral from your primary care physician?

- How and when will you be notified of approval or denial?
- Is there a dollar limit on coverage (such as $100 per visit)?
- Are there copayments? How much are they?
- How are charges paid? For example, is there a usual or a customary charge, is it a percentage, or is there a specific dollar amount?
- Would treatment by some mental health professionals (such as social workers or psychologists at the master's degree level) be excluded by your insurance plan?
- Is there a maximum number of doctor visits on the plan (for example, 25 visits per calendar year)?
- Are any specific diagnoses or types of treatment excluded from coverage?
- Does the provider need to follow a specified treatment plan?

You should be able to find answers to these questions in your insurance handbook. If you cannot find or do not fully understand any information, speak with a benefits representative at work or contact your insurer. If you are not covered or are denied coverage, research other treatment options.

Unanswered Questions at the Doctor's Office

Q For the second time I have gone to a medical appointment and forgotten to tell my doctor about something that was bothering me. Whenever I visit my doctor it seems that he is in such a hurry. I feel rushed. Is there anything I can do to improve the quality of my visits to the doctor?

A Preparing in advance for your office visits will save you and your doctor time and make the visit more constructive. Get organized. Make a list of the issues you want to discuss and questions you want to ask. Be on time. Be clear, direct, and brief. Listen carefully, ask questions, and take notes. Quickly get to the reason for your visit. Try not to get off the subject of your health. Don't be embarrassed to pull out your list—just don't make the list too long. Deal with your present health concerns, not with every health-related event that has ever happened to you. As your questions are answered, check them off your list. Or take a family member or a friend with you to remind you of what you want to ask. If your appointment time is up and you still have unanswered questions, ask if you can have a nurse or a physician's assistant from the doctor's office answer them for you, or if you can call the office later. And before you leave, be sure to ask for any referrals to specialists you may need.

Making the Most of an Office Visit

Here are some useful tips for making the most efficient use of your and your doctor's time at the doctor's office:

- Be on time. If you need to cancel your appointment, give your doctor at least 24 hours notice. If you need to cancel unexpectedly, call and explain the situation. Your doctor and his or her staff will appreciate your courtesy. Also, some offices charge for visits that have not been canceled at least 24 hours in advance.
- Get to know your doctor so you can develop a relationship that leads to mutual trust and respect.
- Do not expect your doctor to be a mind reader. Tell him or her up front what you want to discuss. Explain your problem as clearly as possible. Because your doctor's time is limited and your time is valuable, being direct works to everyone's advantage. Your doctor will appreciate that you

have been considerate enough to take the time to get organized.

- Identify and describe your symptoms clearly. Begin by describing the most serious symptoms. The doctor will want to know when the symptoms first appeared, how often they occur, and how long they last.

- Express observations and concerns about your health. Your doctor will use your input to make an accurate diagnosis. Don't be afraid to talk about your fears or to share advice or information that you have received from friends or relatives or learned from your own research. Your doctor can clarify any misconceptions you may have about your condition, symptoms, or treatment.

- Speak openly and honestly with your doctor. Answer all of his or her questions truthfully and completely to the best of your ability. Keeping information from your doctor can have serious consequences on your health and medical care.

- Be an effective listener. Pay attention to what the doctor is saying. Repeat what your doctor tells you in your own words to make sure you understand what he or she is saying. For example, say something like "As I understand it . . ." or "So what you are saying is . . ." or "In other words. . . . " Don't be embarrassed and don't worry about appearing confused. Your doctor wants to help you understand.

- Use questions to increase your understanding. Asking questions puts you in charge of your health and medical care. If your doctor uses any words or medical terms that are unfamiliar to you, ask for definitions. You need to understand your diagnosis, treatment options, and potential outcomes. Keep the questions as short as possible. No question is too stupid or unimportant to ask. Asking questions now can help you avoid confusion and problems in the future. When you leave the doctor's office, all of your questions should have been answered and all of your concerns addressed.

- Take helpful notes. Bring a notepad and write down the high-lights of your visit, including any special instructions from your doctor. Find out what times you can contact your doctor if you have additional questions after leaving the office.

- Tell your doctor how you feel about your health and medical care. If you are dissatisfied for any reason, let your doctor know as soon as possible. There may be other treatment options available. Discuss the pros and cons with your doctor so you can make an informed decision.

- Ask for referrals. If you feel you need to see a specialist about a specific health problem such as depression, discuss it with your doctor. He or she will refer you to a specialist, such as a psychiatrist, if necessary. If your doctor advises you to see a specialist—for example, an ophthalmologist for a vision problem—be sure to get the names and telephone numbers of doctors whom your doctor recommends. Also, if you are in a managed care plan, make sure the doctor is recommend-ing a doctor who is in your plan. Many health plans require written referrals to specialists.

- Ask your doctor if you can follow up on the phone or by e-mail. If you and your doctor are both online, e-mail may be the quickest and easiest way to exchange information. Be sure to ask your doctor for his or her e-mail address.

Learning about Medical Tests and Treatments

The goal of preventive care is to reduce your health risks to help you stay healthy. Successful preventive care depends, in part, on regular checkups and screening tests. Your checkup involves more than a physical examination and is tailored to your unique health needs. Your doctor will focus on your lifestyle and personal risk factors, and what you can do to stay healthy. He or she will determine which screening tests you need, based on your health risks. Your health risks are determined by a combination of factors, including your age, gender, personal health history, family health history, lifestyle (such as diet, alcohol use, and tobacco use), and any health-related goals you might have (such as whether you are trying to lose weight or quit smoking).

In addition to being a good listener with your doctor and organizing all the questions you have, discuss with your doctor any self-treatments you have used. Your doctor needs to know every method you have tried, regardless of its success or failure in relieving symptoms. Do not hold back information out of concern that the doctor will disapprove. This includes everything from alternative therapies (such as acupuncture or chiropractic), to over-the-counter medications (such as aspirin or cough syrup), to home remedies (such as honey and lemon or chicken soup), to commonsense remedies (such as taking a nap, or soaking in a warm bath).

Once your doctor makes a diagnosis, gather as much information as you can about the recommended treatments for the disease or condition. Start by asking your doctor the following questions:

- What is the name of the treatment? You may want to look for additional information, or talk to other people who have had this treatment. You may be able to find a description of the treatment on the Internet. Ask your doctor if he or she can recommend a Web site that might provide helpful information.

- Why are you recommending this particular treatment for me? Is this the standard, proven treatment for my condition or is it relatively new? Find out if other treatment options are available, what they involve, what their success rates are, and whether you are eligible for them. If you are not eligible, why not? Remember that it is to your advantage to play an active role in the decision-making process.

- What results can I expect? Find out if your symptoms are likely to return.

- What tests will I need, what do the tests involve, what will the tests reveal, how do I prepare for the tests, and when can I expect to learn the results? Preparation may involve taking prescription medications, giving yourself an enema, or other measures. Find out if you need someone to accompany you to the test—for example, if there is a chance you will have anesthesia and not be totally alert afterward. Ask also whether you will need to make follow-up visits, take the test again, or take other tests.

- Will I have to make any temporary or permanent changes in my lifestyle because of the treatment?

Do I Need This Test?

Q I am a man who just turned 30 and I'm uncomfortable with the idea of a "hands-on" prostate exam. I've heard that a blood test is supposed to be more accurate than a physical examination in detecting prostate cancer. Which exam should I have?

A Ask your doctor what test he or she recommends for a person your age. The American Cancer Society (ACS) recommends an annual prostate-specific antigen (PSA) blood test for men over 40 who are at high risk of developing prostate cancer and for all men over 50. These are generally the same guidelines the ACS gives for undergoing a digital rectal examination of the prostate. Therefore, if you have no medical conditions that would require a prostate examination, you probably won't need to have either the PSA blood test or the digital examination for at least 10 years .

Surgery

Of the millions of surgical procedures performed each day across the United States, the majority are not emergencies. Most people have plenty of time to ask the doctor questions that will help them make an informed decision about surgery. If your doctor recommends surgery, ask him or her the following questions:

- Why do I need the surgery? You need to understand the purpose of the recommended surgery—for example, to repair damage, to remove a tumor or a growth, to help diagnose a health problem, to relieve pain, or to save your life.

- What is involved in this operation? Ask your doctor to describe each step of the procedure, perhaps with the help of a diagram.

- Are there different ways of performing the surgery? For example, find out if there is a less invasive technique for this procedure and if you are a candidate for that procedure. And if not, why not?

- What are the potential benefits and risks of the surgery? Any type of surgery has risks, but the benefits should always outweigh the risks.

- What are possible side effects (such as swelling or pain) or complications (such as infection) from the operation? Side effects of surgery usually are predictable, whereas complications are unexpected. Because pain is the most common side effect of surgery, ask your doctor how much pain you should expect and what he or she plans to do to control it.

- What are the success and failure rates of this type of surgery? Ask if the procedure is well established and frequently performed or if it is relatively new or experimental. Also, find out if any special, new, or experimental equipment will be used during the procedure.

- What are the alternatives to surgery? You may be able to avoid surgery by choosing another form of treatment, such as medication. In some cases your doctor may recommend postponing surgery for a specified period of time while he or she monitors your condition (sometimes referred to as "watchful waiting"). If your condition improves, your doctor may postpone surgery indefinitely. However, if your condition does not improve, or perhaps even worsens, immediate surgery may be required.

- What will happen if I decide not to have surgery? Again, you must carefully weigh the potential risks and benefits when making this decision. You need to know if there is a probability that your condition will worsen without surgery or if complications could occur.

- Who will perform the operation? Will your doctor perform the procedure or will he or she refer you to a surgeon? Make sure that the doctor who will perform the procedure is a board-certified surgeon (see page 49). Find out how many times the surgeon has performed this procedure. What were the outcomes?

- Where will the operation be performed? It is important to know whether your surgery will be performed on an outpatient basis (you will not be admitted to the hospital) or if you will have to stay in the hospital overnight or longer. The success rate for a given procedure may vary, depending on where the procedure is performed. Find out how often this procedure is performed and ask about the success rate for the procedure at the designated location.

- Do I need to have any laboratory tests or procedures done in preparation for the surgery? If so, what do the tests or procedures involve? When and where should I have them? Who will perform them?

- What type of anesthesia will I receive for the procedure? With local anesthesia, you will remain conscious, and the specific part of your body that is being operated on (such as your hand or foot) will have no feeling. With regional anesthesia, you will probably be conscious, and a larger area of your body (such as your abdomen) will have no feeling. With general anesthesia, you will be unconscious, and your whole body will be without feeling. Ask about the potential risks and side effects of anesthesia, and find out who will administer the anesthesia and what his or her qualifications are.

- Who will be present during the procedure? What will they do? Will nonparticipant observers be present?

- What is the cost of the surgery, and what is included in this fee? In general, there will be additional charges from the anesthesiologist and the hospital for any inpatient or outpatient care you receive. You will need to find out in advance what portion of these costs your health insurance will cover, and whether you need a written referral.

● When can I expect to leave the hospital, and what is my expected recovery time? When can I return to work? Ask your doctor to describe how you will feel throughout the various stages of recovery. Find out how long you need to wait before you can return to your usual daily routine. Ask your doctor which of your usual activities (including sex) you can perform now and which ones you should avoid, and for how long. Remember that trying to take on too much too soon can lengthen your recovery time. On the other hand, avoiding activities that will help you recover—for example, physical therapy exercises recommended for you—also could delay recovery. Ask your doctor if you will need special care or assistance after you return home. If so, ask your doctor for a referral to a home-care provider, such as a visiting nurse association. Also, find out if you will need any special supplies or equipment to help speed your recovery.

If you do not understand your doctor's answers, ask him or her to explain them in terms you can easily understand. Decide if you need a second opinion. You may want to get a second opinion from another surgeon who is not associated with the first surgeon. Getting a second opinion is a good way to help you make an informed decision. In some cases, depending on the terms of your health insurance plan, you may be required to get a second opinion before the cost of surgery can be covered. In other cases, the cost of a second opinion is not covered by insurance and you will have to pay for it yourself. In any case, be sure that the second doctor receives your records from the first doctor so you do not have to repeat any tests.

Is Your Doctor Board-Certified?

To become board-certified, a doctor must have had at least 7 years of medical training and passed a comprehensive examination in his or her specialty (such as surgery or internal medicine). To find out if a surgeon or any other physician is board-certified, call the American Board of Medical Specialties (ABMS) at 866-275-2267 or, if you have access to the Internet, visit the ABMS Web site (http://www.certifieddoctor.org). You also may access the American Medical Association online doctor-referral service through Doctor Finder (http://www. ama-assn.org). Doctor Finder provides helpful information—such as medical training, specialty, and board certification—on the more than 650,000 licensed physicians in the United States.

Understanding a Diagnosis

A physician makes a diagnosis when he or she identifies a person's health problem and its cause based on symptoms, a physical examination, and the results of any tests. To better understand your diagnosis, ask your doctor the following questions:

- What is the name of my health problem, and what is causing it?
- How will it affect me?
- How long will it last?
- How can my health problem be treated or controlled?
- Can it be cured?
- Will my condition have any long-term effects on my health or lifestyle?
- Can you give me any printed information about my health problem or refer me to an organization that can help me learn more about it?

Your doctor should answer all of your questions clearly and completely. In some cases you may have a difficult time dealing with what the doctor tells you—particularly if it is bad news—and you may have trouble thinking as clearly as you normally would. To help avoid potential confusion or misunderstanding, take notes on what the doctor tells you so you can review the information later and be sure you understand it. Do not hesitate to ask your doctor any questions you may have at this time. And, if you think of additional questions after you leave the doctor's office, write them down and ask them during your next office visit. Or, if you need the information right away, call your doctor and go through your list of questions over the phone. If your doctor's office is online, you might be able to ask your questions via e-mail.

Gather as much additional information about your health problem as possible. The reference librarian at your local library can guide you to a number of helpful resources. After reviewing the information, discuss it with your doctor (or another healthcare provider, such as a nurse) to be sure you fully understand it.

The more information you have about your condition, the better equipped you will be to understand and deal with it. You will then be able to make informed decisions about your medical care and work more effectively with your doctor.

Using Medications Correctly

Your doctor will want to examine you regularly to determine if your medication is working. He or she will also need feedback from you. Think about how you feel since you began taking the medication. Watch for symptoms or side effects and tell your doctor if you are having any problems that could be related to the medication you are taking. He or she can then make any necessary adjustments. Be sure to tell your doctor about any changes you want to make in your treatment plan and why you want to make those changes. Only then can he or she work with you to resolve any problems with your treatment plan and to help ensure that it will be effective. If you decide to stop a medication or to change the dosage on your own, you could affect your treatment in ways that might be harmful.

Drug mistakes are a leading cause of illness and death. To help avoid potential problems, make sure you get specific information about any medication before you take it. Verify any information you get from your doctor with your pharmacist.

When your doctor prescribes medication, be sure to ask him or her the following questions:

- What is the name of the medication (brand name and generic name)? Have your doctor write down the name for you, or ask your doctor to spell it for you as you write it.

- What type of medication is it, and how does it work?

- How will the medication improve or affect my condition?

- How long will it take for the medication to have an effect?

- What are the common side effects of the medication?

- What should I do if side effects occur?

- Could this drug interact with other medications (prescription or nonprescription) I am already taking?

- Can I take the generic form of the medication?

- How often should I take the medication, and for how long?

- When should I take the medication (in the morning, in the evening, before a meal, after a meal)?

- What should I do if I forget to take a dose of the medication? For example, should I take a double dose the next time?

- Should I take the medication on an empty stomach or with food?

- Should I avoid certain foods or alcohol (or beverages such as milk or grapefruit juice), over-the-counter medications, or other substances while taking this medication?

- Should I avoid driving, operating machinery, or engaging in other activities while taking this medication?

- Are there any other special instructions? For example, should I avoid direct sunlight while taking this medication?

- How and where should the medication be stored? For example, does it need to be refrigerated or stored away from moist areas such as the bathroom medicine cabinet?

- How should I take the drug? For example, if it is in pill form, should I take it whole?

The following general points to remember about medication will help you avoid making mistakes:

- Take your medication exactly as directed. Be sure to follow your doctor's instructions carefully. If you do not take your medication exactly as directed, it may not produce the desired effect and can even threaten your health. Don't chew, crush, or break pills unless you have been instructed to do so. If you accidentally skip a dose, be sure to take the next dose at the scheduled time. And never decide on your own to take extra doses of a medication assuming that more medication will help you feel better more quickly; doing so could cause serious problems. Many pharmacies provide information sheets with prescription medications that advise what to do about a missed dose for a particular drug, or you can call your doctor's office and ask.

- Continue taking your medication until your doctor tells you to stop. You may be tempted to skip a dose or stop taking your medication altogether as soon as your symptoms begin to subside and you begin to feel better. However, keep in mind that you are feeling better because you are taking the medication. When your doctor asks you to take medication every day for a chronic or long-term condition such as high blood pressure, it is essential to keep taking the medication to control that condition. Also, with certain medications, such as antibiotics used to treat bacterial infections, you need to use the entire amount prescribed to complete your treatment.

- Store all medications as instructed. As a general rule, store your medications away from heat and moisture, either of which can damage them and alter their effectiveness. Contrary to popular belief, the bathroom medicine cabinet is *not* a good place to store medications. Some medications need to be refrigerated, while others must be kept at room temperature. If you have children in the house, store medications (including over-the-counter drugs) in a locked cabinet or drawer, and request childproof caps for all your prescriptions.

- Never share prescription medication. Your doctor prescribed your medication specifically for you, and you should not share it with anyone. Also, never take medication that was prescribed for someone else. This can be dangerous.

- Check labels, and keep your prescriptions up-to-date. If your doctor wants you to continue taking a particular medication, but the prescription is nearing its expiration date, tell him or her as soon as possible. The doctor can then write a new prescription and you can avoid an interruption in your treatment.

- Discard all medications that are past their expiration date. Because they can lose their effectiveness over time, you should dispose of all medications, including over-the-counter medications, that are past their expiration date. Check the label to determine the expiration date of any medication you are taking. If the expiration date has passed, flush the medication down the toilet, especially if you have children in the home.

It can be easy to become confused about your medication, particularly if you are taking more than one. If you sometimes forget to take your medication, try different strategies to help you remember. For example, make a daily checklist of your medications and doses in the form of a calendar (or mark them directly on a calendar), and check off the dose of each medication as you take it. You can also use an egg carton or a plastic container designed for this purpose to divide up your doses of medication for each day of the week. If you take your medication three times a day, take it before or after each meal. If you take it once a day, take it as soon as you get up in the morning or right before you go to bed at night. In any case, the most important thing to remember about taking your medication is to follow your doctor's instructions. This will help ensure that you get the medication's full benefit, avoid potentially life-threatening complications, and lower your risk of unpleasant side effects.

In general, you can avoid problems with your medication when you remember the following:

- The name (both generic and brand names) of the medication your doctor has prescribed

- When and how to take the medication
- Why you are taking the medication (what it will do for you)
- The possible side effects and what to do if they occur
- How long you need to continue taking the medication

Stopping Medication on Your Own

Q The medication my doctor prescribed is causing unpleasant side effects. Besides, the condition it was prescribed for seems much better. Can I stop taking the medication now?

A Do not stop taking the medication and do not alter the dosage without first talking to your doctor. Making changes in your medication on your own could be harmful to your health. For example, if you have high blood pressure and you stop taking your antihypertensive medication, your blood pressure will go back up. Antihypertensives control, but do not cure, high blood pressure, and you need to keep taking them. If you are taking an antibiotic and do not take the full dosage for the prescribed amount of time, you could make the antibiotic less effective and give the bacteria a chance to grow stronger. If the medication you are taking is causing side effects, your doctor can make adjustments such as changing the dosage or prescribing a different medication.

Making Lifestyle Changes

Some vital factors—such as your blood pressure, weight, and cholesterol levels—should be monitored regularly because of the effects they can have on your overall health. Ask your doctor to check your blood pressure at most office visits, and regularly test your cholesterol, especially if they are at borderline or high levels.

When Your Husband Won't See the Doctor

Q My 50-year-old husband is overweight and a couch potato. He doesn't like doctors, and he hasn't seen our family doctor in more than 10 years. What can I do to convince him that he needs to make (and keep) an appointment for a physical examination?

A You can't force your husband to take care of himself, but you can make helpful suggestions. Perhaps your husband doesn't like your family doctor or had a bad experience with a doctor years ago. Even if you have a managed care insurance plan, your husband has some say in choosing a doctor. Remind him that regular checkups are necessary to test for common disorders such as heart disease. Perhaps your husband is reluctant to hear recommendations from the doctor about lifestyle changes such as losing weight or getting more exercise. Remind him that adopting a healthy lifestyle doesn't mean that he has to stop enjoying life. Besides, he'll feel better and be healthier.

Blood Pressure

Your doctor will check your blood pressure each time you go for an office visit. Maintaining an optimal blood pressure can help prevent serious health problems such as kidney disease, heart disease, and stroke. The best way to keep your blood pressure at a safe level is to maintain a healthy weight, exercise regularly, and follow a healthy diet. Some people may need to take medication to help keep their blood pressure under control.

If you have high blood pressure, your doctor may recommend that you monitor your blood pressure at home. There are many types of easy-to-use home blood pressure monitors available; ask your doctor to recommend one. Your doctor or another healthcare professional (such as a nurse) can teach you how to use your home blood pressure monitor correctly. Keep a record of the blood pressure readings you take at home and bring it with you whenever you visit your doctor.

Weight

Being overweight or underweight can be a factor in a number of health problems, some of which may be life-threatening. Sudden, unexplained changes in your weight (either up or down) can indicate serious problems and should be reported to your doctor at once.

Although your doctor will routinely check your weight when you come for an office visit, it is a good idea to get into the habit of monitoring your weight at home. Ask your doctor what a healthy weight range is for you, and try to keep your weight within that range. If you are having problems losing weight or keeping those extra pounds off, talk with your doctor about developing an effective weight-loss plan. The best way to control your weight is by following a healthy diet and exercising regularly. Weigh yourself once a week, and be sure to keep a written record of your weight.

Cholesterol Levels

Your doctor may monitor your cholesterol—including total cholesterol and the levels of low-density lipoprotein (LDL), the "bad" cholesterol, and high-density lipoprotein (HDL), the "good" cholesterol—for a variety of health-related reasons. Too much LDL cholesterol in your blood can lead to serious health problems such as heart disease, heart attack, and stroke. The best way to control your cholesterol levels is by following a healthy diet, maintaining a healthy weight, and exercising regularly. For help in pursuing a healthy diet, follow the recommendations listed in "Dietary Guidelines for Americans" (see box below).

Dietary Guidelines for Americans

The US Department of Agriculture and the US Department of Health and Human Services developed the Dietary Guidelines for Americans to help you eat right and live a longer, healthier life. The guidelines apply to people who are age 2 and older. By following the guidelines, you can help lower your chances of developing high blood pressure, heart disease, stroke, diabetes, and other common health problems.

- Eat a variety of foods.
- Maintain a healthy weight by combining a healthy diet with regular exercise.
- Eat plenty of whole grains, fruits, and vegetables.
- Choose foods that are low in overall fat, saturated fat, and cholesterol.
- Limit sugar.
- Limit salt (sodium).
- Drink alcohol only in moderation (no more than one drink a day for women and two drinks a day for men).

Exercise

Regular exercise helps keep you healthy in a variety of ways. It strengthens your heart, lungs, muscles, and bones; it helps you achieve and maintain a healthy weight; it helps keep your blood pressure down; and it raises your good cholesterol and lowers your total cholesterol level and your bad cholesterol. Also, regular exercise simply makes you feel good.

Choose a type of exercise that you enjoy, such as brisk walking, swimming, or bicycling. Try to work exercise into your daily routine; exercise on your own, with a friend, or with a group. Start slowly and exercise moderately. Talk to your doctor about developing an exercise program that is best for you.

Tobacco Use

If you smoke, your doctor will recommend that you quit now (see box on page 60). Smoking has been linked to a wide variety of life-threatening diseases, including emphysema, lung cancer, heart disease, high blood pressure, stroke, and kidney disease. When you quit smoking, you significantly reduce your risk of developing smoking-related problems.

Most people who try to quit smoking on their own eventually succeed. The first 4 weeks are the most difficult, but most people lose their craving for tobacco within 8 to 12 weeks. If you have not been able to quit on your own, ask your doctor about using a prescription medication called bupropion hydrochloride or consider using the nicotine patch or nicotine gum. Although both the patch and gum are available over-the-counter, it is a good idea to talk to your doctor so you can learn more about these methods before trying one. Note the warnings on the packaging about not smoking while you use these treatments. Both the patch and gum put nicotine into your system; any additional nicotine might overstimulate your heart and cause serious problems. You also may want to consider joining a quit-smoking group; ask your doctor to recommend one.

How to Quit Smoking

Although it takes a tremendous amount of effort to quit smoking, most people can successfully give up cigarettes. Here are some tips to help you quit smoking:

- Select a date to quit, and stick to that date. Mark your calendar.

- Tell your friends and family about your decision to quit. Tell them you are counting on their support and encouragement to help you succeed.

- Remove all smoking materials (such as cigarettes, cigars, lighters, matches, and ashtrays) from your home, your workplace, and your car. Toss them in the trash.

- Substitute sugarless gum and sugarless hard candies whenever you crave tobacco.

- Drink at least eight glasses of water (8 ounces each) every day.

- Eat low-calorie snacks such as raw vegetables or fresh fruit if you feel hungry. (An increased appetite is your body's natural reaction to quitting smoking.)

- Avoid activities, situations, and places that you associate with smoking. For example, sit in the nonsmoking section of restaurants, and avoid having drinks with friends after work.

- Ask your doctor about using nicotine gum, a nicotine patch, a nicotine inhaler, or prescription medication to help you quit smoking. **Warning:** Continuing to smoke while using some of these methods can pose life-threatening risks to your health, including high blood pressure, heart attack, and stroke.

- Ask a friend or a relative to quit with you or join a quit-smoking group for support and encouragement. Your doctor can recommend a quit-smoking group in your area.

Contrary to what some people may think, chewing tobacco also poses serious health risks, particularly certain forms of oral cancer. If you chew tobacco, your doctor will recommend that you quit now.

Also, in recent years, cigar smoking has increased in popularity as a social activity. Cigars may cause or contribute to lip and mouth cancer.

Alcohol and Other Drug Use

Because alcohol is socially acceptable, people tend to forget that it is a drug. And because it is familiar and widely available, alcohol has greater potential for abuse than any other drug. Alcohol can affect your body in many ways. Like junk food, it provides lots of calories and frequently contributes to weight gain. More serious potential effects of excessive consumption of alcohol include permanent impairment of brain and nerve function, stroke, high blood pressure, heart failure, liver disease, birth defects, increased risk of osteoporosis, and possible increased risk of breast cancer.

Although recent research has shown that moderate drinking may provide some protection against heart disease, doctors do not recommend that nondrinkers start drinking to prevent heart disease. The serious health risks associated with long-term, excessive drinking outweigh any potential benefits.

If you drink alcohol, do so only in moderation. Limit yourself to one drink a day if you are a woman and two drinks if you are a man. A drink is one 12-ounce beer, one 4-ounce glass of wine, or one mixed drink with 1½ ounces of liquor. When you have reached your limit, drink water, juice, or soft drinks instead.

Do you think you may have a drinking problem? Ask yourself the following questions about your use of alcohol:

- Do you lie about the amount you drink?
- Do you feel uncomfortable if you know alcohol will not be available at a social event?
- Do you bring your own liquor along to ensure you can have a drink?
- Are friends or relatives worried about your drinking?
- Do you avoid family and friends while you are drinking?
- Do you like to drink alone?
- Do you drink to relax or reduce stress?
- Do you drink to overcome shyness?
- Do you feel the need to have a drink in the morning?
- Do you drink to help you fall asleep?
- Have you ever had an accident or a close call when you have been drinking?
- Do you forget events or where you were after you have been drinking heavily?
- Have you ever fallen or injured yourself while drinking?
- Have you ever become violent while drinking?
- Do you engage in risky behavior (such as unsafe sex) when you have been drinking?
- Do you become angry or argumentative or regret things you said or did when drinking?
- Have you missed work because you had a hangover?
- Have you been drunk for several days at a time?
- Do you ever feel like you drink too much?
- Do you ever feel guilty about drinking and think about giving up alcohol?
- Do you have any of the physical signs of alcohol dependence (such as shaking, nausea, or vomiting after a night of drinking; red face; enlarged or broken capillaries in the face; memory loss; unsteadiness; or confusion)?

If you answered "yes" to any of these questions, you may have a problem with alcohol, and you may need treatment. Talk to your doctor immediately.

While tobacco and alcohol are the most commonly abused drugs, abuse of illegal and prescription drugs also is a serious problem. Prescription drugs such as painkillers, sleeping pills, and tranquilizers often are abused in combination with alcohol. Alcohol can also interfere with the actions and effectiveness of certain medications, sometimes causing life-threatening adverse effects.

If you think that you, a family member, or a friend may have a problem with alcohol or other drugs, talk to your doctor. Depending on the seriousness of the addiction, he or she may recommend treatment options such as counseling, a support group, or a supervised drug treatment program. You may need to spend several days in a hospital detoxification program.

For additional information, advice, and support, contact the local chapter of Alcoholics Anonymous, the local chapter of Narcotics Anonymous, or the National Council on Alcoholism. Check the phone book for their numbers. And be sure to ask your friends and family for their support in your efforts to over-come your addiction. Admitting that you have a problem and seeking help and support are the first steps toward recovery.

Withholding Information from Your Doctor

Q My job is very stressful, and recently I have been drinking a lot—sometimes five or six drinks a day. I would rather not discuss this with anyone, including my doctor. I have asthma, and the new medication my doctor prescribed is not working well. Could my drinking be interfering with the medication?

A Asthma is a very serious condition that needs to be monitored carefully. You must tell your doctor that the new medication is not working. The alcohol could be neutralizing the effects of the medication or the sulfites (preservatives found in many beers and wines) could be worsening your asthma symptoms. It's essential for you to tell your doctor about the extent of your drinking. He or she will be able to help you deal with both problems.

Clearing Up Misunderstandings

Misunderstandings may occur between you and your doctor just as they may occur in any other relationship. No matter how insignificant the misunderstanding may seem, it is important to resolve it as soon as possible, before it develops into a major problem. Most misunderstandings, when addressed promptly, can be cleared up with a few questions or a brief conversation.

To help prevent a minor misunderstanding between you and your doctor from escalating, keep the following in mind:

- Have realistic expectations of what your doctor can do for you. Do not expect him or her to make house calls or after-hours appointments. Also, do not be offended if your doctor cuts a conversation short or if you have to wait for him or her to return your call; he or she has many other patients and is pressed for time. Sometimes the doctor will ask a nurse in his or her practice to call back with an answer to your question; do not feel slighted, as long as you get the information you need.

- Do not hesitate to tell your doctor if you are having any problems with your treatment. Never wait to say something until your doctor asks you if there is a problem. He or she is likely to assume that everything is fine if you do not say anything. Be your own advocate.

- Let your doctor know if you are dissatisfied with other aspects of your care, such as discourteous office staff, long waits, or problems scheduling appointments. Failing to express your feelings about these seemingly minor aggravations may lead to anger, resentment, and other problems that can interfere with clear communication and have a serious impact on your health and medical care.

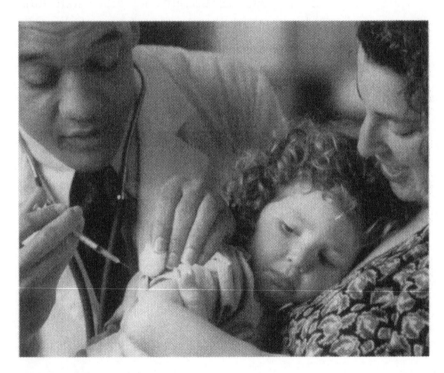

Getting Information for Other People

You may at some point have to accompany another person, such as a child, to the doctor's office. Prepare your child before the visit with a general description of what will occur, especially if he or she is to have a shot. At the doctor's office, you might hold your young child in your lap to help the visit go smoothly. Ask questions and make sure you understand the answers. As your child grows older, encourage a one-on-one relationship between him or her and the doctor.

4

Talking for Others

You seem to be spending a lot of time in doctors' offices these days, but you are rarely the patient. You are there with your child, or your mother or father, and you may be called on to speak on their behalf. The following tips can help you help your loved ones get the most out of a visit to the doctor.

Accompanying Your Child to the Doctor

As a parent, you want to get the best medical care possible for your child, and you want your child's experience getting medical care to be as pleasant as possible. You can do a lot to make going to the doctor a good thing. For children from toddlers to teenagers, the experience of going to the doctor begins at home. Talk about the upcoming visit at least a day in advance, if possible.

When you talk with your child before the visit:

- Be open. No matter what their age, tell your children in advance when they are going to the doctor and why. They need to know what to expect. It helps even young children to know that a "shot" can keep them from getting sick or that a test will let the doctor know which medicine will make them well.

- Be clear. The more you can offer a simple step-by-step description of the visit in advance, the better. Whether it's a finger prick, a vaccine, or a strep test, don't hold back basic information for fear of frightening your child. Children's imaginations can fill any void with scary thoughts.

- Be honest. Never say it won't hurt if it will. Don't say there won't be a shot unless you are absolutely sure about it. If you lie to get through this appointment, you'll have a much harder time going to the doctor with your child in the future.

- Don't be dramatic. There's an important difference between saying "It will hurt for a minute" or "You'll feel a pinch" and saying "It will hurt like crazy!" The expectation to feel pain can actually make the pain worse. Acknowledge that there will be pain or discomfort, but play it down a little.

- Be positive. You're going to see this doctor because he or she can take good care of your child. Your child needs to know that. The doctor wants to help children be healthy and strong. That's true, and it's good to let your child know it too. You may have a long-term, friendly relationship with this doctor, or you may never have seen him or her before. This is no time to appear unsure. Your child needs to know that you trust the doctor.

- Be confident. You may be very worried about what will happen at the doctor's office. You may be squeamish about shots and medical tests. You may be worried that the doctor will discover your child has a serious health problem. If so, tell your spouse or a friend. Don't share your fears with your child. You may find that being confident and calm for your child will actually make you feel less afraid.

- Act it out. For small children, a toy doctor kit and a little dress rehearsal can help ease worries before his or her grand entrance into the doctor's office. Take turns being doctor and patient, taking blood pressure and temperature, looking in ears and eyes. When you are the doctor, praise your fine patient. Be a cooperative and polite patient when you're on the receiving end.

- Don't pry. Assure your preteen or teen that he or she will be able to talk to the doctor, in private, about any concerns he or she may have. Tell your child that you will not become involved unless he or she (and the doctor) wants you to.

At the doctor's office:

- Plan for the wait. The roughest part of a trip to the doctor can be waiting for your name to be called. For small children, bring diapering supplies with you, plus small toys or books and a light snack. Let older children bring books, handheld video games, or anything else they like to amuse themselves with.

- Keep a respectful distance from other children. If your child might have something contagious, try not to pass it around. Don't be embarrassed to ask your child to avoid the toy corner crowd if it looks like he or she might contract something there. If you suspect that your child may have chickenpox or another infectious disease, tell the office receptionist before you arrive. The doctor may want to isolate you and your child in an examining room right away.

- Be prepared. Before you go, think about what questions the doctor will ask and what you want to ask. Make a list to be sure you leave with the answers you need.

- Bring information about any medications. Make a list of all medications your child may be taking, including vitamins and over-the-counter remedies.

- Be ready to clearly describe any concerns you have. Be prepared to answer questions about your child's diet, sleep habits, and behavior, and about when, how long, and how often your child has symptoms.

- Set the tone. Your child learns from you how to relate to the office staff, nurses, and physician. From you, the physician and staff pick up cues about how to treat your child. Friendly is good.

When meeting with your child's doctor:

- Trust your judgment. Your doctor knows about children— but you know your child. Feel free to speak your concerns. If your child eats no vegetables or has terrible tantrums, admit it and get the help or reassurance you need. If there are serious problems at home that affect your child, say so. Your doctor's primary interest is your child's health and well-being.

- Ask any question, no matter how unimportant you think it may be to the doctor. This may be your first child or your third. Still, every child is different, and parents are constantly facing new concerns. Don't hold back a question because you think the question is trivial or because you think you should already know the answer. Your child's doctor will respect your openness and genuine interest in your child's health.

- Make sure you understand every answer. Ask for an explanation if you don't. Ask again if it still isn't clear. If you want more in-depth information, ask for that, too. Your child's doctor talks to many different parents who have different levels of medical knowledge. Let him or her know what you need to know and what your child needs to know. Doctors are used to explaining complicated medical problems and procedures in terms a child can understand.

- Don't be shy about making suggestions. Speak up if you can help things go smoothly. Maybe your child wants to ask something. Maybe your child will sit still while his or her ears and eyes are examined if he or she can sit on your lap.

- Encourage a one-on-one relationship between your child and his or her doctor. Encourage your child to ask and answer questions about his or her body. Your child will feel calmer and more cooperative if he or she feels a sense of control. A trusting friendship between a child and a doctor can be a valuable source of support and guidance in the years ahead.

- Make sure your teen has a general health assessment. Adolescents tend to go to the doctor less frequently than younger children do. Even if this is not your child's first visit to this doctor or office, see that he or she gets a basic health checkup. If you can't fit in an assessment at this visit, schedule one for the next appointment.

- Respect your child's privacy. Teenagers, and sometimes preteens, need the chance to talk alone with a doctor or a nurse.

Encourage your child to feel that he or she can say anything without getting into trouble or worrying about embarrassment. If there's a private conversation between your teen and the doctor, it's important not to pry.

- Compare notes afterward with your child. Review the visit. Listen to your child. Be sure your child understands what happened. If it didn't go well, tell your child it can be better next time. Praise any good behavior. Discuss misbehavior calmly.

If your child is diagnosed with a serious health problem or is facing surgery or a complicated or painful medical procedure, it can be frightening for both you and your child. Here are some tips for helping you make your child's hospital experience less scary:

- First, prepare yourself. Find out everything you can about the procedure, what will happen, and how it will feel. You will be your child's primary source of support and comfort, so you need to feel confident. A solid understanding of the medical situation will help you be the calm parent your child needs now.

- Ask if it will hurt—a little or a lot. Will your child be asleep for the procedure? For how long? Can you be present? Will your child stay in the hospital overnight? Try to think about what your child is wondering, and ask for details you can share.

- Prepare your child. Be open and thorough in the information you provide. Small children understand complicated things better when the learning is hands-on. Role-play or walk some dolls through the experience. Be honest with your child.

- Visit the hospital ahead of time. Many hospitals, and especially children's hospitals, offer a tour and information packet for children who will have surgery or an inpatient stay. Children usually get to wear medical garb, check out medical instruments and surgery suites, and talk to doctors and nurses. Hospital social service departments offer counseling. They can help you locate other resources or support groups for both you and your child. Knowing exactly what will happen—and where—beforehand can make a big difference for everyone involved.

- Teach your child coping skills. Birthing classes teach parents all kinds of coping skills for the pain and fear associated with childbirth. Your child also may need some coping skills to get through a medical event. Learning these skills in advance can help a child feel in control during difficult procedures. Learning to focus, to breathe, to think about good things, to sing, or to squeeze a ball or squeeze a parent's hand are all effective coping skills children pick up easily. For tips on teaching these and other strategies, talk to the hospital staff or your child's physician.

- Read up. Most hospitals provide a packet of basic information to every person entering the hospital for an overnight stay. Ask for one in advance. This information should answer your questions on everything from meal service to discharge planning. The packet should also mention any special services the hospital offers for children, such as tutors to help with schoolwork or craft and play activities.

- Protect your child's rights. Like adults, children have a right to be treated with respect and compassion during their hospital stay. As a parent, you have the right to be fully informed about every aspect of your child's care, and you have final approval of that care. Be sure you know who is treating your child and why. Review the patients' rights information the hospital provides.

● Put your child in charge. Remember that this is your child's visit, not yours. As much as possible, let your child provide the answers to any questions.

If Your Child Has a Disability

Q Two doctors insist that my 6-year-old son needs hearing aids in both ears. They say my son hears only 80 percent of the sounds around him. I cried at the thought that my son will be labeled "different" for having to wear hearing aids. Also, I wonder whether he can cope with the care of these expensive devices, such as taking them out when he goes swimming at day camp and putting them in a protective case. We have an appointment with an otolaryngologist and an audiologist soon. Since my son can hear most sounds, does he really need hearing aids for such a small hearing loss?

A Hearing aids are wonderful technological devices that will help your child do better in school as well as in social situations. It's important that you work with the otolaryngologist and audiologist recommended by your pediatrician to help improve your child's hearing. Most common hearing aids are inconspicuous. A behind-the-ear hearing aid is usually recommended for children because it is safer than an in-the-ear model and is cushioned with a soft material. Also, this type of hearing aid requires fewer repairs than an in-the-ear model. If you present information about taking care of the hearing aids to your son in a positive way, you can help him view the situation as another essential chore, such as brushing his teeth or fastening his seat belt. Most teachers today work with their classes to foster acceptance of children who wear any type of assistive devices, including leg braces or eyeglasses.

Accompanying Your Older Parent to the Doctor

You may at some time need to take your parent to the doctor, perhaps because your parent can no longer get to the doctor's office on his or her own or because he or she wants you there as an extra pair of ears. You know your parent. You can assist him or her by being a companion—and a skilled advocate—at doctors' appointments. Here are some tips to help you help your parent.

Before the doctor visit:

- Make a list of questions together. If possible, your parent should write the list; this is his or her visit to the doctor. If you know of something your parent is worried about but won't ask the doctor, put it on the list.

- Involve the caregiver. If your parent has a full-time or a part-time caregiver, be sure to talk with that person before you make the list. He or she can help your parent think of questions to ask.

- Keep an ongoing list of your own. Pay attention to your parent's medical complaints and worries between appointments. You'll be ready with valuable information when it's time to make a list for the next appointment.

- Find out how much your parent wants to know. If surgery or a major medical problem is to be discussed, your parent may—or may not—want to know the details of a planned procedure or the long-term prognosis. You can make your parent's wishes known and arrange to get the information separately.

- Take all medications with you. The physician can get accurate strength and dosage information from the prescription labels. This is especially important because older people can accumulate a large arsenal of drugs. Also make a list of all the vitamins and over-the-counter remedies, such as laxatives and antacids, your parent takes regularly.

- Make sure you or your parent brings all his or her health insurance cards to the doctor's office.

- Check in with the doctor's office before you leave home. Find out if the doctor is seeing appointments on time and when you should arrive at the office. If you'll have a long wait, it may be easier for your parent to wait at home.

In the doctor's office:

- Ask your parent if he or she wants you to be in the examining room. Don't assume that he or she does. Your parent might not feel comfortable asking you to leave the room; be sensitive to subtle clues. Part of a doctor's clinical skills are to "read" these interpersonal situations. If the doctor suggests you go, excuse yourself.

- If your parent wants you there, be there. Everyone—older people especially—can use a little support and an extra listener by their side at the doctor's office. If the instructions are complicated or if the doctor's news is distressing, your parent may remember very little of what was said. Your parent also may forget important things he or she wanted to say.

- Put your parent in charge, if possible. Let your parent hold the question list and ask the questions. Encourage the physician and the staff to talk directly to your parent. You are there as an assistant, maybe a very active assistant, but one who understands how important it is for your parent to have his or her physician's full attention.

- Help the doctor help your parent. If your mother or father has a hearing problem, ask the physician to speak up and look directly at your parent—not down at the chart—when talking. If your parent forgets a question or doesn't seem to understand an answer, ask the question yourself. Ask the doctor to repeat an answer or to answer more simply until your parent understands it.

- Don't take "aging" for an answer. Few illnesses should be accepted as a "natural part of the aging process." Most conditions now can be treated and cured even in very old people. If your parent's doctor keeps blaming health problems on aging, look for another doctor. If a doctor says your parent is too old for a particular treatment or surgery, get a second opinion.

- Mention major life changes. Death of a spouse, retirement, moving to a new home, illness, loss of a friend, or travel—these and other life events can cause great stress and affect a person's health. Your parent may not want to bother the physician with personal news, but a person's life and health are closely linked. If something important has happened and your parent doesn't mention it, bring it up.

- Pay attention to your parent's feelings. He or she may become overwhelmed by upsetting medical news or feel rushed by the physician. Business as usual may be too fast. Gently let the physician know that he or she needs to explain more fully or to slow down. The physician will appreciate your input.

- Get it in writing. Take notes on your parent's doctor's instructions so you can reassure your parent later that you know exactly what the doctor said to do. Seeing that you're "getting it all down" also may help your parent relax during the visit.

- Get the information your parent needs. If your parent has been diagnosed with a serious disease, ask his or her physician where you can get more information about the disease. If your parent is facing surgery or hospitalization, call the hospital in advance and ask for a patient information packet. Make sure you have plenty of time to read the materials. Finding out everything you can—from when the surgery will be performed, and by whom, to what will be served for meals and when—can help to calm an older person's fears.

- Arrange to get more information if necessary. Sometimes your parent needs to go over something again and there isn't time. Tell the physician. He or she may suggest scheduling another appointment to talk again in a few days. A nurse practitioner or someone on staff may be able to spend more time talking with your parent. There may be a social worker at the hospital who can help. Your parent, just like everyone else, has the right to be fully informed about his or her healthcare. Don't be afraid to ask for the help your parent needs.

- Make sure your parent has a geriatric assessment. If this is a new physician for your parent, or if your parent goes to the doctor only when he or she has a specific problem, ask to schedule a geriatric assessment, which is a general health checkup geared to the health concerns of older people.

- Get information for any questions that linger. After the appointment, go over everything that happened and exactly what the doctor said. If your parent seems upset by the information, talk about it again later, when he or she has had some time to relax and think.

- Respect your parent's right to privacy. Your parent is an individual, and some medical questions are not your business. Offer and be prepared to leave the room anytime your parent wants to talk alone with the doctor.

- Don't downplay your parent's concerns. What you might dismiss as an imagined or exaggerated problem may be something real, something the doctor can treat. Let the physician make the evaluation.

- Treat your parent with respect. In the physician's office or the hospital, remember that you help define who your parent is and how he or she should be treated. Caring for an older parent who is easily confused can be difficult even under the best circumstances. But in the rush of activity surrounding a medical situation, everyone can get edgy. Slow down, be patient, and be considerate of your parent's feelings. Show the respect to your parent that you want others to show him or her.

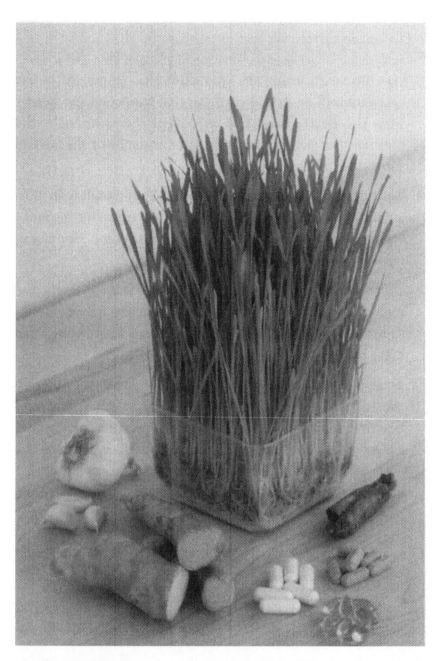

Being Open and Honest

When your doctor asks you about medications you are taking or alternative treatments you may be trying, be honest. Your doctor needs to know about all medications you are taking, including vitamin and mineral supplements and herbal remedies. In some cases, herbal remedies and other over-the-counter health products can interfere with the effects of a medication your doctor has prescribed. And some herbal remedies can be harmful.

5

Talking about Sensitive Subjects

Every person, from time to time, has a medical problem or issue he or she would rather not discuss, even with a trusted doctor. Maybe you think you'll just have to live with it. But you shouldn't—it's better to be honest about lifestyle issues such as drinking or smoking. Straightforward discussions with your doctor may disclose a simple solution to your problem. No matter how unusual or embarrassing you feel your problem is, you won't be the first to mention it. Doctors are skilled at treating all kinds of problems. Once you open up about a problem, you'll find your doctor reassuring and able to help.

Keep in mind that patient-physician communication is confidential. Unless you give your permission, your doctor will not share anything you say with anyone else. However, some medical information must be reported to state or federal authorities. For example, child abuse must be reported to local child welfare agencies. Gunshot wounds must be reported to the police.

Top Hard-to-Talk-about Topics

The following medical conditions or health concerns are the most difficult subjects for people to discuss with their doctors:

Sexually transmitted diseases

Homosexuality and bisexuality

Sexual problems

Alcohol dependence

Drug addiction

Family violence

Depression

Incontinence

Self-treatments

Dissatisfaction with treatment

End-of-life healthcare issues

Statistical data on sexually transmitted diseases must be reported to the public health department.

You came to the doctor with a simple sore throat or a headache. Maybe you're feeling fine, and this is your first meeting with a new doctor. So why all these embarrassing questions about how much you drink and smoke, your diet, your job, your worries, your parents' health, your personal relationships, and health problems you've had in the past? Your answers to questions such as these help your doctor understand you and your healthcare needs. Answer truthfully. Don't worry about being judged. The more open you are with your doctor, the more he or she can do to help you. A thorough health review can enable your physician to make important connections leading to a diagnosis that might otherwise be overlooked. And, in an emergency, a physician who has access to your medical history is equipped with life-saving information.

Sexually Transmitted Diseases

Sexually transmitted diseases (STDs) top the list of hard-to-discuss topics. STDs are among the most common infectious diseases in the United States; four STDs rank in the top ten reportable diseases in the United States. About 15 million new cases of STDs occur each year in the United States, and the number is rising. People of every age, race, background, and economic level contract STDs.

STDs require immediate treatment. With early treatment, most STDs can be cured. If you are concerned that you might have an STD but you can't bring yourself to talk about it, the following points should convince you to make an appointment now:

- Even if you have no symptoms, you could have an STD. Many people, especially women, do not have any noticeable signs of disease when they first contract an STD. Symptoms that do appear may look like signs of another, less dangerous condition, even a common cold. Only medical tests can determine whether you are STD-free.

- Early diagnosis can make all the difference. Almost all STDs can be treated and cured if detected in the early stages. Left untreated, some of these diseases can become life-threatening. Some STDs can cause infertility, cervical cancer, damage to the heart and central nervous system, or even death. These risks are greater for women because they may not realize they have an STD until more serious symptoms arise.

- Untreated, some STDs can be passed from a mother to her fetus during pregnancy or to her baby at birth. Some STDs can cause miscarriages, premature births, and death of the newborn. Babies may be born with pneumonia, eye infections that can cause blindness, mental retardation, or damage to the nervous system. With proper medical care during pregnancy, a baby can be born healthy.

- You may unknowingly give the STD to someone else—and get it back again yourself. Having had an STD does not provide immunity to it. You can get some STDs over and over again. Both you and your partner may need treatment to cure the infection.

- New tests and new treatments for many STDs are available. Don't hesitate to see your doctor about an STD because you've heard there's no cure. This is a very active area for medical research. New medications to effectively treat and cure STDs are being developed all the time. Vaccines currently are being developed to prevent several STDs, including acquired immunodeficiency syndrome (AIDS), chlamydial infections, genital herpes, and gonorrhea.

- Some STDs put you at increased risk of contracting the human immunodeficiency virus (HIV), the virus that causes AIDS. Having an untreated STD, such as syphilis, makes you more likely to contract HIV if you are exposed to it.

- For HIV and AIDS, early diagnosis and treatment are essential. While there is currently no cure for AIDS, new, powerful drugs taken together can greatly enhance the quality of life and prolong the life of a person with AIDS. Because these treatments are most effective when started early in the course of the infection, it's essential to be tested right away if you think you may have been exposed to HIV. Researchers continue to search for new drugs that are more effective against HIV over the long term.

How should you talk to your doctor about an STD?

- Phone the doctor's office and ask to speak to a nurse or a physician's assistant. Give the reason for your call. The nurse or physician's assistant may be able to address some of your concerns and give you practical advice over the phone right away. He or she also can help get you an earlier appointment if necessary.

- At the time of your appointment, remind the nurse or assistant about the reason for your visit. If you find the topic embarrassing, say so. Be honest about your problem and about your feelings so your doctor understands how best to help you feel comfortable.

- Be direct and open with the doctor in asking and answering questions. The doctor will ask questions about your symptoms and about your sexual practices to help him or her diagnose and treat your problem and help you to stay healthy in the future.

- Volunteer information the doctor hasn't asked about if you think it might be important. For example, you may be pregnant, you may have infected another person, or you have had this or another STD before. Telling the doctor can help ensure that you get the help you need.

- Ask the "silly" question that is bothering you. And try to clear up any wrong information you have gotten such as "You can get this STD from a toilet seat." Your doctor has heard it before and will give you the correct information.

If you have been diagnosed with an STD, follow your doctor's instructions exactly. Take all the medication prescribed to be certain you are cured. Avoid all sexual activity during treatment if you have been told to do so. If you don't agree with your doctor's recommendations or if you think you'll have problems following them, discuss it with your doctor before you leave the office. If your doctor gives you a prescription for a drug you've taken before and had problems with, tell him or her about it. Don't just decide not to fill the prescription; the doctor can probably substitute another drug.

What if you have no special reason to suspect you have an STD? You should still ask for an STD screening test as part of your regular checkup if you are sexually active and not in a mutually monogamous relationship. Most doctors routinely provide STD screening tests to their patients who are at increased risk of STDs.

If you suspect you may have an STD, see your doctor. If you don't have a doctor, contact the National Center for HIV, STD, and TB Prevention (see page 161). It offers free information about STDs and has lists of private physicians and clinics throughout the country that provide treatment for STDs. You can get information without leaving your name.

Homosexuality and Bisexuality

Many lesbians, gay men, and bisexuals avoid seeing the doctor and, when they do, they may not get satisfactory healthcare. Fear of being judged often makes them reluctant to seek healthcare. Even when they have a primary care physician, they sometimes don't disclose their sexual orientation for fear that the information might negatively affect their healthcare.

If you are homosexual or bisexual, make sure you're talking to the right doctor. A good doctor for you is one who treats you respectfully and who is knowledgeable about gay and lesbian health concerns. You need a doctor you can trust and talk to openly and honestly. Talk about your sexual orientation with the doctor you have now. Be open and forthright about getting the healthcare services you need. Simply saying you are gay, lesbian, or bisexual may not tell your physician enough about your health risks. Be frank about your sexual behavior and lifestyle so the doctor can assess the impact it can have on your health. For example, all women need to have regular gynecological examinations. If you are gay, lesbian, or bisexual, and not in a mutually monogamous relationship, you need to be screened for STDs.

If your doctor makes you feel uncomfortable, change doctors. Ask your homosexual or bisexual friends for recommendations. Your health insurance may require you to select a physician from its list of primary care providers. Remember that as a managed care consumer you have the right to be treated with respect by your physician and the right to change physicians if you are unhappy with your care. When selecting a new doctor from within the system, ask if he or she is experienced in gay or lesbian healthcare. If you don't like the response, select a different physician. Sometimes your primary care physician needs to refer you to a specialist. If a specialist does not treat you respectfully, alert the referring physician. You should also report the incident to your health insurance company.

Sexual Problems

Sexual problems are common in both women and men. Some sexual problems have a physical cause, while others may result from psychological inhibitions or childhood sexual abuse or are rooted in aspects of a couple's relationship. The most common sexual problems are lack of desire, difference in sex drive between sexual partners, difficulty achieving orgasm, painful intercourse, premature ejaculation, and erectile dysfunction.

Because of the personal nature of sexual relationships, most people are reluctant and embarrassed to discuss the subject with anyone else, including their doctor. But most sexual problems can be treated successfully. For this reason it's important to talk to your doctor about any problems you are having. He or she can rule out a physical cause or treat it.

For example, if you are a woman and your lack of sexual desire is caused by a decline in hormones at menopause, your doctor may prescribe estrogen in hormone replacement therapy. In men, most cases of erectile dysfunction (ED)—the inability to achieve an erection or to sustain an erection for sexual intercourse—result from physical problems. Diseases such as diabetes, kidney disease, atherosclerosis, or multiple sclerosis; injuries; hormone imbalances; alcoholism; smoking; drug addiction; and stress can cause ED. The effects of some prescription medications account for nearly one of four cases of ED. Treatments for ED can range from changing a medication or taking a smaller dose to making simple lifestyle or diet changes. Ask your doctor about the newer medications for treating ED.

If your sexual problem stems from your relationship with your partner or another emotional issue, your doctor can refer you to a qualified sex therapist for counseling. Keep in mind that no matter how self-conscious or embarrassed you feel about your problem, your doctor has heard it before. The more open you are with your doctor or therapist, the more successful your treatment is likely to be.

Alcohol Dependence

If you think you have a problem with alcohol, you may need help. Maybe you drink a little too much, maybe a lot too much. Or you only drink now and then, but overdo it sometimes. If you have any concern at all about your drinking, you need to talk to your doctor. You should also talk to a doctor if you are concerned about the drinking of your spouse, another family member, or a friend. The doctor will give you an objective opinion, plus help if it's needed.

You don't have to be dependent on alcohol for it to harm your body. Heavy drinking can cause liver disease and can contribute to some cancers. Even small amounts of alcohol are harmful during pregnancy; fetal alcohol syndrome is the number-one preventable cause of mental retardation in the United States. A pregnant woman who drinks also runs the risk of having a miscarriage.

If you have ever driven while drunk, you need immediate help. Don't fool yourself about your level of tolerance for alcohol. There is no safe level of alcohol consumption for drivers. No one should ever drive if he or she has been drinking. And don't ride with drivers who have been drinking.

Insist on the help you need. If your physician dismisses your drinking problem, repeat that you need help. He or she should respond not just to the amount you drink, but also to your concerns about it. Ask about support groups or other resources that can answer your questions and offer assistance.

Your physician treats many people who have problems with alcohol. Don't be afraid to ask for help:

- Be specific. Tell your doctor how much you drink, how often, when, and with whom.

- Be honest. Don't underestimate; you are there to get help, not to fool the doctor.
- Describe your diet and exercise habits.
- Discuss how drinking is affecting your personal and professional lives.
- Ask for help. Your doctor can refer you to counseling, a rehabilitation program, or a support group.

If you are reluctant to talk to your physician, call a local hospital and ask for information about services in your area. Look in the phone book under "Alcoholism" for local chapters of Alcoholics Anonymous (AA) and other alcohol-dependency support groups. Rehabilitation and support services all protect their clients' right to privacy.

If you think someone you love has a problem with alcohol:

- Share your impression that something is wrong. Tell him or her that you are worried. Keep your tone conversational— don't be argumentative, and don't raise your voice. Above all, try not to lecture.

- Mention changes you have noticed in the person's appearance and behavior. Bring up any of the signs (see page 62) that you have noticed.

- Be optimistic. Stress that medical help and other types of support are available and that these strategies have helped thousands of people successfully stop drinking. Suggest that the person ask his or her doctor to be a partner in helping to solve the problem.

- Be supportive. Show the person you want to help with your continued concern and support, but emphasize that he or she needs more help than you alone can give.

Drug Addiction

Just like alcohol, drugs can harm your body and destroy your life. In addition, taking illegally obtained prescription drugs or street drugs is against the law. If you are using illegal drugs, you need help. Talk to your doctor. Remember that anything you say to your doctor is confidential. He or she is experienced at helping people with substance abuse problems of all kinds. Drug addiction, like alcohol dependence, is a medical problem. Trying to break a serious addiction on your own can be physically dangerous and may be impossible. With support from your physician and the right treatment program, you can recover fully.

Drug and alcohol rehabilitation programs that can help you start on a new life often are covered by health insurance. Check your coverage to see what is available, but be ready to pay for treatment yourself if necessary.

Family Violence

If you are the victim of family violence, or domestic violence, you may be confiding in friends or relatives but keeping the situation from your physician. In reality, your doctor is the first person you should tell. The doctor's office is a safe place where you can get treatment for injuries and help in handling a current crisis. If you are the aggressor, your physician can help you find support to prevent recurring violence.

Don't wait for your physician to ask you about violence in your family. Although most primary care physicians ask their patients about domestic violence if they are treating them for injuries, few doctors ask a new patient about domestic violence at the first appointment. Fewer still mention the topic during routine office visits. Fear of offending a patient makes this a tough topic for physicians to introduce. However, every physician has seen family violence and its physical and emotional consequences more than once. Half of all injuries to women seen in hospital emergency departments are the result of domestic violence, and more than half of rapes of women over age 30 are committed by their partners.

Don't be offended if your physician asks you questions about domestic violence. Domestic violence affects people in all racial and socioeconomic groups. Stress is often the trigger that brings violence into formerly secure and loving homes. If your physician questions the source of an injury or asks if there is any trouble at home, be truthful. Your physician wants to help you, not judge you.

When a child is hurt, the child's safety is all that matters. Take your child to the hospital or see your child's doctor right away. Be honest about how the injury occurred. Doctors and hospital staff are legally required to report all suspected cases of child abuse, whether a parent admits to the abuse or not. For a gunshot or stabbing wound, or other clear indication that a violent crime has been committed, a physician or a hospital is legally required to report the injury to the police. If you are involved in family violence of any kind, it's essential to get help immediately.

Depression

Depression is not a personality weakness, nor is it something you have to live with. It's normal to feel sad sometimes, especially when bad things happen. The loss of a loved one, problems at work, an illness, a major disappointment, or other unhappy events can bring on temporary feelings of despair. However, not all sad feelings are normal, and not all sadness goes away. If you have a depressed mood that lasts more than 2 weeks, arises for no apparent reason, or interferes with your ability to function, you need to talk to your doctor.

Some people hide their unhappy feelings from their physician because they see unhappiness as a sign of personal weakness. Others become accustomed to feeling bad most of the time and think of it as their natural state, not worth mentioning to a doctor. Maybe you aren't sad but you feel irritable, or you're tired all the time. You may feel sick. Maybe you bounce between feeling energized and feeling listless. All these can be signs of depression and a reason to seek help. Medical treatment can cure depression or significantly reduce its symptoms in more than 80 percent of all cases. Without treatment, depression may linger for months or years and can become increasingly serious and more difficult to treat.

Clinical depression is a common medical condition that results from an imbalance of chemicals in the brain. Every year one of ten American adults experiences depression. Depression affects people of all ages, from the very young to the very old. Children who are depressed may be dismissed as moody or difficult. However, childhood depression is an increasingly common problem that can lead to a lifelong condition or to suicide at a young age. Old age is often a time of great personal loss and physical limitations. Some sadness is natural, but lingering sadness is not. Depression can be successfully treated in older people.

To get help for your depression, see your primary care physician first. Sometimes depression is a symptom of an underlying disease or is caused by a reaction to a medication. Your physician will rule out these possibilities before referring you to a mental health professional for treatment. Treatment for depression usually involves medication or psychotherapy or both. The combination of medication and psychotherapy usually is the most effective. Nearly all cases can be treated successfully.

Depression usually is treated with medications called antidepressants. Antidepressants do not artificially elevate mood but relieve depression by altering the balance of the chemical messengers in the brain that stimulate mood. You may need to take an antidepressant for several weeks before you notice a difference or you may need to try different medications. Some people need to take more than one antidepressant at a time to improve their condition.

Although most side effects of antidepressants usually subside in a few weeks, tell your doctor if you experience any. Some common side effects of antidepressants include constipation, drowsiness, dry mouth, headaches, insomnia, or nervousness. Meet with your doctor regularly while you are taking antidepressants so that he or she can adjust the dosage of your current medication or prescribe another antidepressant if you experience side effects.

Antidepressants are not addictive, and their benefits can last long after you stop taking them. Although they are usually taken for only about 6 to 18 months, it is important not to discontinue taking them prematurely. Continue taking the medication until your doctor tells you it is time to stop.

In psychotherapy, or talk therapy, you discuss your feelings and how they are affecting your life. Psychotherapy involves meeting with a psychiatrist (a medical doctor who specializes in treating mental disorders) or a clinical psychologist or a clinical social worker (nonphysician experts educated in counseling and behavior management therapies). Any of these therapists can help you learn how to manage or change your feelings over time. Talking through your feelings to change your state of mind can bring about positive physical changes in your brain chemistry.

In an emergency:

- If you have considered suicide, tell your physician immediately and get help. Go now to your doctor's office or a hospital emergency department and ask for help.

- Take talk of suicide seriously. Despair may cause people to do things they would never normally do. Pay attention if a friend or a family member—especially a child—mentions suicide, even in a joking way. Get help for him or her as soon as possible.

- Stay. If you think someone is in danger of hurting himself or herself, stay by his or her side until you have delivered him or her into safe care at a hospital emergency room. You could save a life.

Incontinence

Incontinence is the involuntary loss of urine from the bladder or the inability to retain stool in the rectum. Urinary incontinence is common among older people, especially older women. Although the condition has different causes, most cases can be treated successfully.

Talking about Personal Matters with Your Doctor

Q I have problems controlling my bladder. I have gone to the doctor a number of times about the problem, and she has been very helpful. She has recommended a series of exercises and other techniques to help correct the problem. My condition is much improved but it doesn't get any easier to talk about it. How can I get over my embarrassment?

A Most talk between a doctor and a patient is of a personal nature. Try to remind yourself before each visit that even if you are uncomfortable your doctor is used to talking to her patients about matters that seem very personal. Your situation is common and your doctor has discussed it with many other patients with the same problem.

Urinary Incontinence

Urinary incontinence is a common but distressing and sometimes disabling medical condition. One of three women over 60 and many men have incontinence at some time in their lives. But because most people incorrectly think that incontinence is untreatable, they never mention the problem to their physician. Instead, they struggle to deal with it on their own.

Living with incontinence is not easy. Trying to avoid embarrassing accidents in public means using disposable pads and padded undergarments. It may mean restricting activities. Urinary incontinence is the number-one reason why elderly people are forced to give up independent living and move into assisted-living facilities.

No one should simply accept incontinence. In the past, this condition may have been something a person was forced to live with, but it no longer is. More than 80 percent of all cases of incontinence can be cured, allowing people to return to full, active lives. In other cases, the symptoms can be relieved and the condition made much more manageable.

Treatments for incontinence range from simple exercises to diet changes, drug therapies, hormone replacement cream, or,

Types of Incontinence

Incontinence has several forms, each identified by how the person experiences the problem:

- *Stress incontinence* is the involuntary leaking of urine caused by increased pressure inside the abdomen during activities such as coughing or sneezing or high-impact exercises such as jogging.

- *Urge incontinence* is the involuntary leaking of urine after a sudden, uncontrollable urge to urinate caused by an involuntary contraction of the bladder muscle.

- *Mixed incontinence* is a combination of stress and urge incontinence.

- *Overflow incontinence* is the periodic leaking of urine when the bladder fills to a point at which it can't hold any more.

in some cases, surgery. Urology is the medical specialty that deals with incontinence and other problems of the urinary tract. Call your primary care physician to discuss the problem; he or she may refer you to a urologist.

Before your appointment, begin keeping a daily log of your problem for at least a week. When does the leaking occur? How much leaking do you have? How much warning do you get before you leak urine? Knowing exactly how you experience the problem will help the urologist determine the possible causes and find the best treatment for you.

An important part of your office visit will be the interview with the urologist. Your description of the problem, along with lifestyle and diet information, may point to a simple solution. The urologist may perform minor medical tests for incontinence, and he or she may recommend one or more outpatient hospital procedures to help make a diagnosis.

If the doctor recommends specific exercises, be sure you understand exactly how to do them. Ask for written instructions. If the problem persists, tell him or her. A number of good solutions to this problem are available, and your physician may recommend another treatment.

Fecal Incontinence

Fecal incontinence—the involuntary loss of fecal matter, or stool—is an even more difficult problem to live with or talk about than urinary incontinence. While not as common as urinary incontinence, fecal incontinence, too, is a condition that many people try to hide when they should be looking for help. Feelings of embarrassment make many people with fecal incontinence withdraw from family and friends.

Getting help for fecal incontinence begins with a call to your primary care physician. He or she probably will refer you to a gastroenterologist—a doctor who specializes in disorders of the colon and rectum. Fecal incontinence has a variety of causes, including an underlying disease or injury. The condition can be successfully treated, sometimes with measures as simple as reducing stress, increasing exercise, or changing your diet.

Your doctor also can help you find a support group for people who are dealing with fecal incontinence. In these groups, people who have fecal incontinence share practical advice about dealing with the condition and give each other understanding and encouragement.

Self-treatments

Physicians know that the healthiest people are those who take an active interest in their own well-being, who ask questions, and who take responsibility for their health. More and more people are reading scientific articles about medical care, searching the Internet, networking with other people who have the same medical condition, and trying all kinds of therapies on their own. Walk into a health food store or stroll down the vitamin aisle in virtually any drugstore and you'll see high-potency multivitamins targeted to every stage of life, plus an alphabet of individual vitamins that address various health issues. You'll find herbs, teas, lotions, creams, drinks, purges, and peels.

Don't expect your doctor to be shocked if you're thinking of trying something on your own. More and more physicians are recommending alternative therapies such as acupuncture, meditation, or massage as helpful additions to traditional healthcare. However, always tell your doctor about any alternative therapy you are using. Some alternative therapies are dangerous. Other alternative therapies may be harmful by keeping you from seeking the medical care you need. While one in three Americans has used an alternative therapy, 80 percent of them fail to tell their doctors about it.

To be on the safe side:

- Report to your doctor all the vitamins and herbal supplements you take, and the amount of each. Some vitamins are stored in the body for long periods and can be toxic at high doses. Some vitamins and supplements can interfere with the body's ability to absorb prescription medications.

- If your diet is unusual, describe it to your doctor. Radical diets can be harmful and may be dangerous for people who have certain medical conditions. Also, the presence or absence of some foods in your diet can affect the potency of prescription medications you are taking.

* Be sure to tell your doctor about any over-the-counter drugs and health food or home remedies you are using. Some of these can be toxic when combined with prescription medications and may cause allergic reactions.

* Before starting a strenuous exercise program, check it out with your doctor.

* Talk to your doctor about your past—or planned—use of alternative therapies. Bring along to your appointment scientific articles or other information about an alternative treatment you want to try. Your doctor can tell you how a particular therapy might work in conjunction with your regular healthcare. Think twice about seeing an alternative therapy provider who does not want to work with your physician.

If some therapy you have tried has worked wonders for you, tell your doctor. He or she may want to share your good idea with others.

Dissatisfaction with Treatment

You might be dissatisfied with your doctor's treatment but you aren't sure why. You may not want to admit that you didn't follow your doctor's instructions. Perhaps you didn't take the medicine exactly as prescribed, or you stopped taking the pills when you began to feel better or because the medication had side effects. Maybe you missed several doses in a row, or you took more of the medication or less than you should have. Maybe you never even got the prescription filled.

Tell your doctor. Medicines taken for too brief a time or at the wrong dosage can do more harm than good. If the medication had unpleasant side effects or was too expensive, your doctor may be able to prescribe an alternative. If you don't take a medication exactly as indicated, your doctor cannot correctly assess its effectiveness in treating you. Tell your doctor as soon as you discover you have a problem with your treatment; don't wait. The sooner the problem is cleared up and you start a treatment you can stay with, the sooner you'll get better.

Your main concern should be getting the help you need. Your doctor can provide guidance or direct you to other sources of support for help in achieving your long-term health goals. If you are not happy with the care you are receiving, talk to your doctor. Quality healthcare is based on two-way communication between you and your doctor. You need to be able to talk to your doctor about your health concerns openly and honestly, and you should expect to be treated with respect. If you feel your doctor isn't listening to you or doesn't understand your problem, say so.

Ask for clarification if you have trouble understanding what your doctor tells you. Like any interaction, a doctor-patient relationship can take a bad turn if there is a misunderstanding. A frank discussion of your concerns may be all that is needed to set things right. A very fine doctor is not a good doctor for you if you don't feel you can talk to him or her about all your health concerns. Sometimes a busy doctor will ask a nurse or a physician's assistant to handle a patient's needs or answer health-related questions. If you have tried talking to your doctor or his or her assistant and still feel uncomfortable or unsatisfied, you might consider changing doctors (see Chapter 1). Also, you should probably consider changing doctors if you have questions about the quality of care you have received, and these issues are not resolved.

If you have serious concerns about a physician's care, you may need to file a complaint. First, ask your health insurance provider if it has a patient advocate who can talk with you about your complaint, your rights, and any actions you should take. If the problem occurred during a hospital stay, your first recourse is to talk to a hospital patient advocate. If the issue is not resolved to your satisfaction, contact your local county or state medical society for help.

Access to New Treatments

Q I am 45 years old and have recently been diagnosed with breast cancer that has spread to my lymph nodes and liver. My doctor has recommended treating my advanced stage of cancer with high doses of chemotherapy followed by a bone marrow transplant. I called my health insurance plan to see if it would pay for this treatment but found that this type of therapy, specifically the bone marrow transplant, is not covered. They told me the bone marrow transplant is considered experimental. What do I have to do to get my health insurance plan to pay for a bone marrow transplant?

A Set up an appointment with the transplant center or hospital through your doctor immediately. Have the transplant center contact your insurer to review the request and resolve any questions. Your doctor should forward a letter to the insurer, along with copies of studies and articles that support the transplant recommendation. The studies should be very recent and emphasize safety and effectiveness, but especially should underscore how the therapy is accepted in the medical community. Also send a copy of a second opinion. This should resolve the question of a therapy being "investigational" or "experimental." Get the most recent copy of your insurance plan booklet and gather any other healthcare insurance information you can from your employer to back up your claim. However, if you have to go to court to appeal denial of coverage, the reasonableness of the insurance company's decision is usually the issue, not the appropriateness of the therapy. ▓▓▓▓

End-of-Life Healthcare Issues

Planning for future medical care, particularly when you might not be able to make your own decisions, is called advance care planning. Think of advance care planning as a form of preventive care. Consider carefully the difficult decisions that may have to be made on your behalf and discuss them with your family, acknowledging that you can change your mind at any time. The process of advance care planning helps you identify and document your preferences concerning medical treatment. Failure to make your wishes known may confuse your physician and cause disagreement between your physician and your family.

When to Start Planning

Many people think that it is their doctor's responsibility to initiate advance care planning. But don't wait until your doctor brings up the topic. This planning is easiest to accomplish when you are in good health. Decisions that have to be made when a person faces a life-threatening illness or major trauma can be difficult and complicated.

Don't be surprised, however, if your doctor is the one who brings up the topic. Federal law requires that Medicare and Medicaid beneficiaries who are admitted to a hospital or skilled nursing facility be asked if they have advance directives if they are receiving hospice or home health benefits or if they are enrolled in a managed care plan. Advance directives are written instructions concerning medical care that is to be carried out when a person has lost the ability to make his or her own decisions. Physicians have a legal and professional responsibility to comply with a person's advance directives.

End-of-Life Healthcare Decisions

Q I have just learned that my elderly mother is terminally ill. She has told me many times that she does not want to be kept alive by machines. What can I do to ensure that the doctor and the hospital respect her wishes?

A While your mother is still well enough to make her own legal and health-related decisions, contact her doctor and a lawyer to discuss the possibility of issuing advance directives. Advance directives are legal documents that provide guidance and instructions for healthcare providers to ensure that any healthcare decisions that are made on a person's behalf are consistent with his or her wishes. Advance directives may include a healthcare proxy (durable power of attorney for healthcare), a living will, and do-not-resuscitate (DNR) orders.

Benefits of Advance Care Planning

In addition to the sense of control and peace of mind it can bring you, advance care planning has other important benefits. It is helpful to those close to you because they may have to make decisions about your medical care and related matters if you cannot. It can help strengthen your relationship with family members and with your doctor. Collaborating with your doctor on your plan will ensure that your wishes for your care are spelled out in your medical records. This communication process will help you see if you and your physician agree on important care issues.

Advance care planning also helps you clarify your personal values and goals. You will identify what you would and would not like to have done in various situations. You will identify who you would like to make healthcare decisions on your behalf in case you cannot speak for yourself. You will be exercising your right to participate in and direct how your healthcare needs will be addressed if you ever lose the ability to make decisions.

Helpful Terms

- *Advance directives* are instructions spelling out a person's wishes regarding medical care in case he or she has a physically or mentally disabling illness or accident and cannot speak for himself or herself. This is an all-inclusive term used to describe the terms below.

- *Medical directives* are sets of instructions based on possible illness scenarios, medical care goals, and treatments.

- *Instructional directives* are directives for care that usually are recorded in letters to a person's doctor and family members.

- A *healthcare proxy (durable power of attorney for healthcare)* is a person authorized to act on behalf of a person who is unable to direct his or her care plan.

- A *living will* is a legal document that specifies the kind of treatment a person wants when he or she is dying, such as attempting or not attempting resuscitation, or using or not using a ventilator or other heroic measures to extend a person's life if his or her prognosis is poor.

Children and Advance Care Planning

The thought of planning for your child's future medical care is a parent's worst nightmare. But children and parents may still benefit from such a plan. Advance care planning ensures that a child's parents have discussed in detail a child's treatment options should the child ever be in a critical-care or crisis situation. Remember, the purpose of advance care planning is to be prepared.

Choosing a Healthcare Proxy

Designating a person to be your healthcare proxy (durable power of attorney for healthcare) is a worthwhile initial step in your advance care planning. It is helpful to involve him or her in subsequent conversations with you and your doctor. Because the proxy is empowered to make decisions for you when you are incapacitated, he or she should be someone you trust. And he or she must be willing and able to carry out your wishes. The best proxy for you might not be a family member or spouse because a close family member may be overly influenced by his or her emotional attachment to you on the one hand or by the burden of care on the other. The decisions that have to be made are sometimes too difficult for an individual who is close to the person. The key is to select someone who will honor your instructions and make decisions according to your shared values.

Considering Care and Treatment Options

When evaluating your care and treatment options, consider all the possible healthcare scenarios with your doctor. For example, what would you want done if you were in a coma and not expected to recover? Your doctor will suggest a number of possible courses of action. He or she may also suggest possible interventions (such as a ventilator for artificial breathing) or treatments (such as antibiotics) for various situations and ask you how these fit into your goals.

Think about your values and beliefs when you are faced with a life-threatening condition. Take time to reflect on your treatment options, and talk them over with your family and others who might be affected by your decisions. Your doctor will discuss your decisions with you before anything is finalized to be sure that they are medically feasible and to make certain all possibilities have been discussed. Advance directives are not permanent and can be revised at any time.

Getting Your Advance Directives in Writing

Some people want their healthcare proxy to make decisions for them without providing the proxy with specific instructions. Most people want to make their own decisions and view their proxy as a backup. It may be helpful to provide written instructions about future situations and interventions that you do not want performed on your behalf.

The wording of healthcare proxy or living will documents varies slightly among the 50 states, but any document that clearly represents your wishes is legal. A worksheet that you have used to review the process can be formalized and used as the official document. Keep a copy of your advance directives, give a copy to your proxy and family members, and have your doctor put a copy in your medical records. You also may have a copy sent to a hospital or regional or national health center. Advance care planning is not a onetime event. It is an ongoing process that needs to be reviewed and updated regularly. Don't forget to keep your doctor, proxy, and family members informed of any changes you make in your advance directives.

Organ Donation

The need for donated organs and tissues for transplants far exceed the supply. The waiting lists of people who would benefit from receiving a transplanted organ are long. Many will die without one. Most families who have donated a loved one's organs find comfort in knowing that they and their loved one have given life or health to another person. For example, 80 percent of people who receive a donated kidney are alive at least 5 years later. Available donor organs are matched to recipients based on a number of factors, including similarity of blood and tissue type, medical urgency, the length of time they have been on the waiting list, and where they live (transplants are more available in some areas of the country than in others).

If you want to donate your organs after your death, make your intentions clear to your relatives and sign a donor card. You can obtain information and applications from a local hospital, healthcare organizations such as the American Red Cross, or your local library. You can also find information on the Internet. For example, at the federal government's Web site (http://organdonor.gov) you can download a copy of a donor card to fill out. In addition, it's a good idea to indicate your wish to be an organ donor on your driver's license. Ask your secretary of state's office how to do so.

You should know, however, that even if you have signed a donor card, all states require the permission of a close relative (spouse, adult child, or adult sibling) before your organs can be donated upon your death. For this reason it is especially important to make your wishes clear to your family.

Organ donation does not conflict with the beliefs of most religions or affect funeral practices, including an open casket. The organs are removed from the donor's body immediately after his or her death. In ideal circumstances, the organs are removed while a person (who has been medically certified brain-dead) is still connected to a heart-lung machine, which circulates blood and oxygen to the organs to keep them viable for transplantation. The organs are removed quickly, refrigerated, and transported immediately to a designated hospital, where they are transplanted into a waiting patient.

The donor's family does not pay any of the costs related to the donation of organs and tissues. All expenses are paid for by the organ recipient's private health insurance or by Medicare or Medicaid.

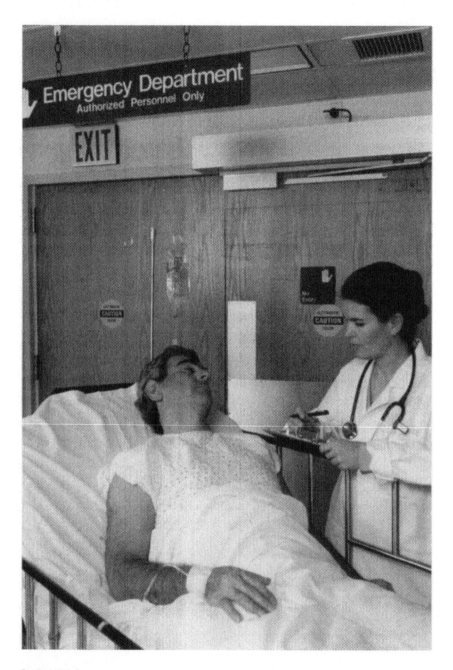

Be Prepared

Emergencies are never planned, but you can be prepared in case you or a loved one is in an emergency situation. For example, know what hospital you should go to if an injury occurs at home. Be ready to provide hospital personnel with a list of medications you are taking and any allergies you have. If you have a chronic illness such as type 1 diabetes, you should always wear an identifying bracelet or other indicator of your illness. Carry your health insurance card with you at all times.

6

Special Situations

You may, at some time or another, have a medical problem that your primary care physician is not familiar with or experienced in treating. In this case, he or she will refer you to a doctor who specializes in an area outside of his or her field of expertise. Or you may need to have surgery or accompany your child to the emergency department. The information in this section will help you deal with these situations, communicate your concerns, and get the medical care you need for yourself or a loved one.

Do I Need a Specialist?

Q I have had the same doctor for many years but have recently been diagnosed with multiple sclerosis (MS). I don't think my current doctor is up on the latest treatments for my condition, and I am concerned that I am not getting the best possible care. I like my doctor and don't want to hurt his feelings by going to another doctor. Do you think I need to change doctors?

A If you have other ideas or thoughts about treatments or philosophies you have researched, bring them to the attention of your doctor. Give the doctor a chance to read and research them, and explain what he recommends and why. If you still aren't assured of your doctor's expertise in treating MS, ask him or her for a referral to a neurologist who specializes in MS. Because you seem comfortable with your physician in general, you may decide to see a specialist for your MS in addition to your regular doctor for your general healthcare needs.

Specialists and Subspecialists

Within some areas of specialization are subspecialties. Specialties and subspecialties were created to address the complexities in the practice of medicine and the intensive training required to be expert in a particular branch of medicine. For example, within the specialty of emergency medicine, a physician may be further certified in the subspecialty of pediatric emergency medicine. Within the specialty of orthopedic surgery, a surgeon may be a subspecialist in hand surgery. An obstetrician-gynecologist may be a subspecialist in reproductive medicine or gynecological oncology.

A physician certified in a medical specialty has completed the traditional 4 years of medical school, followed by up to 7 additional years of intensive study in an area of specialization. He or she has passed a rigorous certification examination in that field.

To keep abreast of current research and updated treatments and procedures, many specialty boards require specialists to take periodic recertification examinations.

The 24 Fields of Medical Specialty

The American Board of Medical Specialties recognizes the following 24 fields of medical specialty:

- Allergy and immunology
- Anesthesiology
- Colon and rectal surgery
- Dermatology
- Emergency medicine
- Family practice
- Internal medicine
- Medical genetics
- Neurological surgery
- Nuclear medicine
- Obstetrics and gynecology
- Ophthalmology
- Orthopedic surgery
- Otolaryngology
- Pathology
- Pediatrics
- Physical medicine and rehabilitation
- Plastic surgery
- Preventive medicine
- Psychiatry and neurology
- Radiology
- Surgery
- Thoracic surgery
- Urology

Identifying Specialists

Your primary care physician may be a specialist who is board-certified in family practice or internal medicine. Other specialists who serve as primary care physicians include obstetrician-gynecologists and pediatricians. Make sure that any physician you see for expert care is certified in his or her specialty. Specialty and subspecialty board certification is your assurance that the physician is qualified and trained in this particular area of medicine.

To find out if a medical specialist or subspecialist is board-certified, or to locate a certified specialist in your area, contact the American Board of Medical Specialties' free Certified Doctor Verification Service (866-275-2267).

Coordinated Care and Other Health Services

You may be referred to a specialist by your physician, or you may select a specialist yourself. In either case, you should give the specialist the name of your primary care physician and ask that information about your care be sent to him or her. Your doctor needs to be aware of all your medical treatments to provide well-integrated care for you.

Your physician also may refer you to a variety of related healthcare specialists who are not physicians. Psychologists, rehabilitative therapists, speech therapists, chiropractors, optometrists, podiatrists, nutritionists, birth instructors, and a host of other nonphysician specialists provide additional services that can help round out a treatment plan. Always feel free to ask any healthcare provider about his or her training and background. Your insurance plan may cover some of these services but not others, or provide coverage only when certain conditions exist. Ask in advance about your benefits.

Getting a Second Opinion

There are many good reasons to get a second opinion. In many cases an insurance plan will require a second opinion before approving elective surgery or other procedures. If your plan requires a second opinion, it will pay for it and probably can help you find a physician for it.

You may be the one who wants a second opinion. Don't be shy about asking for a second opinion. This is your health. Sometimes an insurance company will pay for a second opinion even if it does not require it. If you are eligible, Medicare will cover the cost of a second opinion. Consider getting a second opinion whenever you want one, even if you have to pay for it yourself. Another opinion may convince you that the first physician's diagnosis or recommended treatment was wrong, and you will avoid an unnecessary medical procedure. If the second opinion agrees with the first, you will feel reassured.

When to get a second opinion:

- *When you have been diagnosed with a life-threatening or rare disease.* You need to be sure that the diagnosis is correct before proceeding with treatment. Symptoms of serious or rare disorders can be surprisingly similar to symptoms of less serious conditions.

- *When a treatment plan is proposed for a serious or rare disease.* Make sure that your physician is recommending the best course possible for treating the disease. A serious disease may require a prompt, aggressive approach.

- *Whenever elective surgery is proposed or any other invasive or expensive procedure is part of the plan.* In an emergency, there is no time for choice. When you're planning surgery, you have time to consider alternatives. Any surgery carries a degree of risk. Make sure the benefits of the surgery are greater than the risks involved. Ask both your physician and another physician the following questions: What do you recommend? Why do I need this surgery? What are the benefits of the surgery? What are the risks? What if I don't have this surgery? Are there other, less invasive, options? What is your experience performing this surgery?

- *When you aren't sure about the physician.* Talk to another doctor. The diagnosis and treatment plan may both be right for you, but what about the physician? You want someone who is well qualified and has lots of experience performing this surgery or procedure. Ask about the doctor's qualifications. Find a skilled surgeon who has a solid track record performing this surgery.

- *Anytime you want another opinion.* It is important for you to get the assurance you need before accepting a diagnosis or starting on a course of treatment. If your instincts tell you to verify what you have been told, do it. You, not the doctor, have primary responsibility for your healthcare.

How to get a second opinion:

- *Ask your physician for a referral to another doctor.* Physicians are accustomed to referring patients for second opinions, especially since many insurance plans require them. Make sure your physician sends copies of your records to the physician who is giving the second opinion.

- *Find a doctor yourself.* If you choose to seek a second opinion on your own, you can find a specialist by checking with a nearby hospital or medical school or going to a physician who has been recommended by someone you know. When you choose a physician for a second opinion, he or she will need all the information available to make an informed opinion. Call the first physician and ask that a copy of your records be sent to the second physician's office.

● *Ask an expert.* Locate a medical center that specializes in your disease and ask your physician to refer you to that center. Or call the center yourself and find out how to get an appointment. See the section on rare diseases (page 128) for ideas on finding a qualified medical center.

Do I Need a Second Opinion?

Q My doctor has recommended surgery, but I have heard that my condition can be successfully treated with medication instead. How can I be reasonably sure that my doctor is recommending the best course of treatment for me?

A You may want to get a second opinion. Getting a second opinion from another physician who is not associated with your doctor will help you make an informed decision. Some health insurance plans require second opinions before they will cover the cost of surgery, while other plans neither require nor cover the cost of second opinions. If your insurance plan doesn't cover the cost of the second opinion, you will have to pay for it yourself.

At the Hospital

A hospital can be an overwhelming place, with doctors, nurses, and technicians arriving in your room unexpectedly or wheeling you off through a maze of floors and rooms for tests and treatments. Fortunately, there is a master plan to all your hospital care. The better you understand the plan, the more at ease you will feel during your stay.

Who Is in Charge?

Anytime you are a patient in a hospital, one doctor assumes overall responsibility for your care. The doctor who is in charge of your care throughout your hospital stay is referred to as your attending physician.

If you are admitted through the emergency department, the emergency physician will admit you and name the surgeon, obstetrician, internist, or other physician who will provide care during your stay.

Should your primary diagnosis change during your hospital stay—if while in the hospital for one health concern you are found to have a different or more serious medical problem—a different doctor may become your attending physician. The attending physician is the person in charge of all of your care when you are hospitalized—from the meals you are served to the actions of every hospital staff member who participates in your treatment. When the nurse brings a medication or says that it is time for you to try walking after surgery, he or she is following your attending physician's orders. Lab technicians, respiratory therapists, medical students, internists, and residents who appear in your room are all there following your attending physician's orders. The attending physician will select other specialists to consult with on your case as needed. He or she also will call your primary care physician when you are admitted and discharged and may consult with your primary care physician during your stay.

Who Is Treating You?

When you are in the hospital and you don't know who the person is who is treating you, you should ask:

- Who are you?
- What are you here for?
- Did my attending physician refer you?

Physicians and other healthcare providers should volunteer this information when they arrive in your room. If they don't, it's important to ask. If you don't understand why a test is necessary, ask about it. If a nurse brings you a medication you didn't expect, don't take it until you're sure it's correct. If you have questions about someone's training and qualifications, ask. It is not rude to ask questions. Patients have the right and the responsibility to be fully informed, active participants in their healthcare. In most states, hospitals are required to post a Patients' Bill of Rights.

While your attending physician directs your care, a team of physicians may be involved in carrying out his or her directions. Various specialists may be consulted on your care. At a research or teaching hospital, you may receive care from physicians at all levels of training, from senior residents to interns and medical students. Registered nurses (RNs) may be assisted by licensed practical nurses (LPNs) or licensed vocational nurses (LVNs) and nursing assistants.

Asking Questions

Your attending physician may make hospital rounds to check on patients early in the morning or late at night. When he or she arrives at your room, you may be asleep, or on another floor having tests or therapy. The attending physician will look at your chart, or hospital medical record, to review any test results and check your vital signs (temperature, pulse, and blood pressure), which the nurse has taken and recorded on the chart.

Hospital stays are short now, and many tests and procedures may have to be done in a single day. When you do see the doctor, you may find it hard to remember all your questions or exactly what the doctor said. Have someone listen with you. When your physician is explaining important information, have a family member or friend with you to hear it. If no one can be there, ask a nurse to stay and listen. Did your doctor say you should be ambulating? That means it's time to walk. That you're afebrile? This means you don't have a fever. If you are having trouble understanding your doctor, ask him or her to explain again, or ask someone, such as a nurse or physician's assistant, to explain it to you later.

Don't worry if you forget. The chart the nurse uses to record your vital signs is also the place where the physician writes down all his or her orders. Did your doctor say you should get up and walk this evening? Can you have visitors today? What did he or she say about the results of your blood test? The things your doctor told you, or didn't get a chance to tell you, will be recorded in the chart. Ask the nurse to look up the information you need.

Reaching the Doctor

The nurses or residents (if you are in a teaching hospital) are your best line of communication with your attending physician. They can reach the doctor quickly. If you are concerned about something and the answer isn't in your chart, they can page the doctor in the hospital or call the doctor's home or office for you. If a question is important to you and a nurse or a resident doesn't call your doctor for an answer, call him or her yourself. You have the right to be fully informed about and involved in your care.

When You Are Unhappy with Your Care

If you are unhappy with your care, tell the nurse. Tell your attending physician and tell your primary care physician. Talking openly about the problem to your nurse or doctor should be all that is needed to change the situation. If you object to the treatment you received from any member of your healthcare team, express your concerns. You have the right to request that an individual not attend you.

If the problem is not resolved or if you have serious misgivings about your care, contact the hospital's patient advocate. You'll find the advocate listed in your hospital information packet. Or use the hospital's hot line. Every hospital is required to provide a special hot-line number that patients can call to address their complaints directly to the hospital's administration. Feel free to make a complaint. Quality healthcare is your right. The American Hospital Association officially adopted a Patients' Bill of Rights more than 25 years ago. Hospitals across the United States adhere to these principles in providing care. Look in the patient information packet you received when you entered the hospital. Your hospital's own printed version of these rights should be there. If not, ask for one.

Your rights include:

- The right to considerate and respectful care
- The right to understandable information concerning diagnosis, treatment, and prognosis
- The right to appropriate pain assessment and management
- The right to know the identities of everyone involved in your care
- The right to make informed decisions about your care and to refuse care

- The right to privacy
- The right to review your medical records
- The right to consent to or decline to participate in a research study
- The right to be informed about hospital resources for resolving disputes or grievances

With these rights come responsibilities. Among other things, the American Hospital Association document points out that patients must provide accurate information about past illnesses, hospitalizations, medications, and other matters related to their health status. It also states that patients can ask questions and request more information about their medical condition and treatment if they do not fully understand what they have been told by their physician or another healthcare professional. Patients can tell their physician if they will not be able to follow their treatment program.

Leaving the Hospital

The amount of discharge planning required when you leave the hospital is determined by the complexity of your case, your age, and your home situation. For example, a fit 30-year-old man who is going home to his family after minor elective surgery may simply be told to check in with his physician's office in 2 days or to make an appointment to see his doctor in a month. But a frail 80-year-old woman who lives alone and is leaving the hospital after being treated for a broken hip will need plenty of well-coordinated medical care and social services when she is discharged.

Your discharge, like your hospital stay, is supervised by your attending physician. When you are ready to go home, someone familiar with your care—your physician, your nurse, or a special discharge nurse—will carefully go over your discharge orders with you. Your discharge plan will have been developed by the physicians, nurses, therapists, nutritionists, and other healthcare professionals who were involved in your care during your hospital stay. If you require at-home care, they will work with the social worker and home healthcare specialists who will be involved in your care.

You should be involved in the planning process so you won't have any surprises. Get a written copy of the instructions and make sure you fully understand what you are to do, who will be there to help if ongoing care is needed, and whom you should contact if you have questions or concerns once you leave the hospital. If possible, plan for your ongoing care before you are admitted to the hospital. This is the best time to ask for the help you may need. Maybe you live alone and will not be able to care for yourself during your recovery period. Perhaps you will need a wheelchair or home healthcare services or rehabilitative care. If you ask for help in advance, the transition from hospital to home can be a smooth one. Be frank about your home situation and the reasons why you feel you will need assistance. Your primary care physician may know you well, but your attending physician may not have seen you before this hospital visit. If you don't tell your attending physician what you need, he or she can't help you.

Talk to your physician about discharge needs when you schedule a hospital stay. Call the hospital social services department as soon as you know you will need help. A social worker will be happy to talk with you in advance about discharge planning. Also, talk to your nurse. The nurse will ask about discharge plans and your home situation as part of your initial assessment when you first come under his or her care. If you are concerned about your recovery period, talk to the nurse about it during your stay.

It is the patient's responsibility to ask in advance how any medical condition or procedure will affect his or her life. Find out what to expect during your recovery and in the future. Ask specific questions. Will you be able to care for yourself? Will you be able to care for your family? Will you need a wheelchair? Will you require a special diet or physical therapy? Will a nurse visit you? If so, how often?

Hospitalization, medical complications, and the need for ongoing support services can arise unexpectedly. Fortunately, the hospital staff is skilled at handling surprises. Call the social services department as soon as possible during your hospital stay and keep them updated if your needs change.

In an Emergency

In an emergency, every minute counts. If someone is bleeding heavily, is not breathing, is having a seizure, is unconscious, or has a severe burn or other serious problem, call 911 or your local emergency number. If it's faster, take the person to the nearest hospital or medical center yourself. Don't think about whether the person's insurance will be accepted at this hospital or whether he or she can afford the bill. Just go.

For true medical emergencies, hospitals are required to treat all patients regardless of their ability to pay. Once you or a loved one are stabilized and can be moved, you or the hospital can request transportation to a hospital where your medical care will be covered by your health insurance. Generally, insurance companies approve emergency care at the nearest hospital. They usually offer a 24- to 48-hour grace period for reporting emergency department treatment. If you have questions about coverage, talk to the clerk who took your identification and insurance information when you arrived. Once the initial crisis has been taken care of, it is time to think about where you are and, if you need further care, where you should be. Don't be afraid to ask questions.

When you're dealing with a not-so-urgent emergency, such as a broken bone or minor burn, and you have a choice of several hospitals nearby, take a minute to think about which hospital emergency department you should go to and why. Is there a children's hospital nearby? A hospital or medical center with a plastic surgeon on call? Maybe you want to head for the hospital where your own doctor is on staff or a hospital covered by your insurance plan. A little planning ahead and a slightly longer drive now may turn out to be worthwhile.

What to take to the emergency department:

- *Any medications you are currently taking.* Throw all current medication containers in a bag and take them with you to the hospital. The prescription labels will tell the emergency department team exactly what you are taking, the dosage, how often you take it, and when you took the last dose.

- *Information about any allergies.* Doctors need to know about all allergies because of possible allergic reactions to medications that are used in an emergency department.

- *Someone who knows what happened.* Doctors are better able to provide effective treatment when they know how an injury occurred or have a description of the first symptoms of an emergency medical condition.

- *Insurance card and identification.* These are needed for hospital paperwork and billing.

Go to the emergency entrance of the hospital, not the lobby. Even if the problem is not life-threatening, use the emergency entrance. Park your car in the area marked for emergency patients. Don't block the emergency entrance; make sure you are in a designated parking place. Ambulances need space to back up to the emergency entrance and you don't want your car to be in the way. However, if it's a life-threatening emergency, you should drive right up to the door. Make sure the person is safely handed into the care of the emergency department medical team and then go move your car. Some hospitals provide valet parking for emergency patients.

Emergency departments operate on a worst-case-first basis. When you arrive, you will see a nurse who will determine the urgency of your case. To limit the confusion and protect the privacy of their patients, some hospitals have rules strictly limiting who can be with a patient during treatment. Others will let one or two people stay with a patient. Even parents may be asked to remain in the waiting room in cases of extreme emergency or during some medical procedures. If you are the patient and have someone with you in the waiting room, tell the nurse. He or she can make sure your friend or family member gets updates on your condition. If you need some support, a nurse can ask the person to join you.

Before you leave, the emergency department staff is likely to call your primary care physician while you are being treated. If they don't, you can ask them to call and give your doctor a report. A doctor or a nurse will go over discharge instructions with you. Make sure you understand what they tell you; ask for a written copy of the instructions.

When It's Your Child

If your child is being cared for in the emergency department, you are no doubt nervous and upset. But to help your child get the best care possible, try to do the following:

- *Bring all pertinent information with you.* Bring any medications your child is taking. It's a good idea to keep a copy of your child's immunization record where you can find it quickly. For example, in an emergency, knowing when he or she had the last tetanus shot can prevent your child from having a shot he or she doesn't need.

- *Be calm.* In times of crisis, children mirror—and magnify— their parents' emotions. If you look frightened, your child will be terrified. If you act hostile toward the hospital staff, your child will be afraid of them—and mistrust you when you hand him or her into their care.

- *Ask questions.* Keep your voice calm to reassure your child, but ask questions and pay attention to what happens. Don't be intimidated by your surroundings. Ask that your child's doctor be called. If you want a plastic surgeon or other specialist (such as an ear, nose, and throat specialist or an oral surgeon) to stitch up a face wound, ask for one. If you don't understand why a doctor or a nurse is doing something, ask. If you don't get the answers you need, ask again.

In the Waiting Room

Depending on the emergency, you may or may not be able to remain with the person you brought in. It's best to stay out of the way and trust the medical staff to do their job. If you are facing an emergency alone and feel overwhelmed by the experience, you can get help and support even while you are sitting in the waiting room. Ask for a hospital social worker or chaplain to be with you.

No news is not bad news. Emergency departments can become very busy very quickly. The medical team may not have sufficient time or staff to keep you informed. Not getting an early report is not necessarily a sign that things are going badly. Keep in touch with the nurses' station for information. Stay out of any "Do Not Enter" areas.

Rare Diseases

You or a member of your family has been diagnosed with a rare disease. What should you do? Here are some steps that may be helpful:

- *Double-check the diagnosis.* Rare diseases may be rare, but their symptoms often aren't. You may have this disease, or something much more common. Don't be sure of the diagnosis until one or more other physicians have examined you.

- *See an expert.* The initial diagnosis may have come from your primary care physician or from a specialist. Make sure you are examined again by a physician who has experience and expertise treating this disorder.

- *Go to the best.* Ask your doctor about seeking a second opinion and exploring other options. Your physician should be able to help you find a physician or a medical center that has experience treating people with your disorder.

- *Ignore the odds.* This disease may be so rare that only one in a million people gets it, or it may be so lethal that only 5 percent survive. Don't be lulled into inaction or scared by statistics—they don't tell you anything about your unique case. You could beat the odds—many people do.

- *Be positive.* If a physician says there is nothing he or she can do for you, find another physician. For rare disorders of every kind, new treatments are being tried, and research continues. You need to connect with a physician who is up-to-date with the latest treatment options and able to help you.

- *Double-check the treatment plan.* Once the diagnosis of a rare disorder has been made, be sure you understand the treatment plan. Ask another physician who is a specialist in this field what he or she would recommend, and compare plans. Get a third opinion if necessary. Keep asking questions until you are convinced you are getting the care you need.

- *Triple-check extreme measures.* Is major surgery involved in the treatment plan? Intense rounds of chemotherapy? A procedure that seems radical or experimental? You need to know in advance whether this is the best course for you.

When the going gets rough during treatment, it will help you to know that what you have chosen is the right treatment for you. Ask the following questions and make sure you understand the answers:

- Why is the treatment or procedure being done?
- What can I expect?
- What other options do I have?
- How much time do I have to think about this before making a decision?
- Is this the standard treatment for my disorder?
- Where can I get more information about this procedure?
- Is there a less invasive procedure we can try first?
- What will happen if I don't have this procedure?

For more information about your disorder, contact the National Institutes of Health Office of Rare Diseases (see page 166), which has extensive data on a number of rare diseases. No matter how rare your condition, you are likely to find a doctor who specializes in it and can provide treatment to people like you. Someone is likely to be doing research on your disorder, and people are probably undergoing experimental treatments at research centers.

Ask your physician or local hospital for information about a support group of people who have your disorder. Look up the disorder on the Internet. You may find a national support group. Other people with the diagnosis also may be looking for support. But keep in mind that not everyone experiences the same disorder in the same way or reacts in the same way to "cures" or treatments.

When living with a rare disorder, it can be comforting to talk with someone who shares your problem. You can get a lot of support and practical advice from other people who are involved in the same struggle. Also, by networking, you can share information on research studies and the latest medical advances. But be skeptical about any advice you get from anyone other than a doctor who has seen you. Support groups, Web sites, and other online sources are helpful for gathering information, but for your medical care, or that of a member of your family, you may be compromising your health if you accept recommendations from anyone other than your doctor.

Talk about your disorder with friends and acquaintances. You never know who can connect you to a support group or a new research study. Talk to your representative in Congress about your disorder and the need for new research. Publicity for a disorder and public pressure for a cure can help bring in money for research, as has happened with breast cancer and AIDS.

You hope for a cure and a return to a normal life. Although there might not be a cure for your disorder, there is likely to be research to find a cure or a method of prevention. Volunteer to participate in a study. You can at least have the satisfaction of doing your part in the battle against this disorder. By volunteering for research, you also can receive new treatments before they become available for general use. Read the next section to find out about volunteering for research.

Participating in Clinical Trials

Sometimes the best course of action is to try something new. As a volunteer in a clinical trial, you have the chance to try a therapy while it is still being studied. A clinical trial—also called a clinical protocol or clinical research—is a research study designed to help doctors and scientists understand, diagnose, prevent, treat, or cure a disease. The main goal of a clinical trial is to scientifically test the value of a specific drug, device, or therapy for a specific disease.

The first thing to know about a clinical trial is that it is research, and it is a trial. The treatment being studied may prove to be effective or not effective. The treatment may be found to have unpleasant side effects. You are a participant, not a patient, in the research. The medical treatment you receive is based on the requirements of the research protocol, not on your individual needs as a patient. When you are considering joining a clinical trial, find out exactly what your participation will mean, what possible risks and benefits it presents, and how this clinical trial compares with other options you have.

Clinical research is divided into three phases. The stage at which you enter a research project will determine how much is already known about the treatment you are to receive and how you will participate in the study.

Phase 1 clinical trials test how much of a drug can be tolerated without causing unacceptable side effects. The first few participants are given a low dose of the drug. The next groups get increasingly higher doses. Phase 1 participants are studied for side effects, not for how well the drug works against their disease. A phase 1 trial is likely to offer little or no benefit to a participant.

Phase 2 clinical trials come after a drug's effective dose has been established and its side effects are known. In these trials, many more patient volunteers are given the drug. Participants are studied to see how well the drug affects their bodies and how well it works against the disease.

Phase 3 clinical trials compare the new drug against a drug that is already being used to combat the disease. Some participants are given the new drug, and some are given the established drug.

In a clinical trial, a new drug may be tested against other drugs or against a placebo, which is an inactive substance made to look like the drug being studied. To protect the accuracy of their results, drug trials are randomized, meaning that whether volunteers get the drug or a placebo is decided by chance. You may be in a single-blind study, in which you do not know which drug you are receiving but the people carrying out the study do. Or you may be in a double-blind study, in which neither you nor the doctors or nurses caring for you know which drug you are receiving.

The Benefits of Participating in Medical Research

For many people, participating in a clinical trial is a way to help find a cure for a condition they or a family member has. For some people this participation is their only chance for a treatment that may help cure their condition. Here are some more of the benefits of taking part in a research study:

- You will be involved in up-to-date research on the treatment of your disorder. If a drug is proven to be highly effective and safe during a clinical trial, the protocol may be broken and all participants, including those in the placebo group, will be offered the treatment.

- Your health will be very closely monitored throughout the study period. You will receive more frequent, thorough examinations and medical tests for your condition than you would receive in standard medical practice. All these tests give your physicians and you a much more detailed understanding of your condition.

- Your welfare is important. If a therapy is not in your best interest, you will be removed from the study. Researchers will then discuss treatment options with you and your primary care physician.

- You may be able to participate from home. Even federally funded research is often performed at scattered sites around the country. Your local hospital, your physician, or a nearby medical center may be taking part in a study.

- There is no charge for your care if you are participating in a government-funded clinical trial. Taxpayers' dollars cover the costs of government-funded research, even if it involves a lengthy hospital stay or years of ongoing care.

The Risks of Participating in Medical Research

Although participating in clinical research can be beneficial, it also can carry some risks. Because the treatment under study may not have been proven safe, it could cause undesirable or potentially harmful side effects. Consider the following when you are thinking about participating in a clinical trial:

- A clinical trial is an experiment. The new drug or therapy under research in a clinical trial may prove not to be effective at all in the treatment of your disease. Or it may have very unpleasant side effects.

- You may not be getting any treatment at all. If you are in the placebo group of a double-blind study, you may not be getting the experimental treatment. Taking a less effective but proven drug under your primary physician's care might be a better choice than being in the untreated group in a research project.

- The research is not tailored to your needs. You must adhere to the study's protocol, taking the drug exactly as required and following all of the required conditions, even though you might benefit personally from a different treatment strategy.

You have the final say in what happens to you by giving your fully informed consent. All research subjects must be fully informed and consent freely to participate in a clinical trial. This means that you must be told—in terms you can understand—all the specifics of the research protocol. You must understand what the treatment is, how the study will be conducted, and what the potential benefits and risks are for you.

You will receive a written consent form that carefully spells out everything you need to know to make an informed decision about participating in the clinical trial. You also will be told about the protocol and have the chance to ask questions before you sign on as a research subject. The researchers who are involved in the study are likely to be enthusiastic about their work and about the potential benefits of the therapy they are testing. Before volunteering for the study, it is a good idea to get a second opinion. Talk to a specialist who is not involved in the project about the risks and benefits and about what participating in this protocol can mean for you. You have the responsibility to do what is best for you. Before the clinical trial begins and at any point during your treatment, you have the right to ask questions—and the right to be fully informed.

At any time, for any reason, you can stop being part of a clinical trial. You can quit in the middle of a course of treatment, or refuse a specific treatment or procedure that is part of the research. However, understand that by refusing to participate in part of the study you may be disqualifying yourself from participation in other parts of the study. Before you begin your participation in a clinical trial, your right to leave at any time should be clearly explained to you. This is an important safeguard for research subjects. Physicians and nurses involved in the study should be willing to talk with you about other treatment options.

If you have any problems or concerns about a clinical trial, you can file a complaint at any time—before you enroll, during the trial, or after your participation is completed. Address your concerns to the Office for Human Research Protections of the Department of Health and Human Services (see page 148).

Finding a Clinical Trial

For the most complete listing of clinical trials in all areas of medicine, visit the Warren Grant Magnuson Clinical Center clinical trials' Web site (see page 149). Here you can search for clinical trials by diagnosis or symptom, by the institute of the principal investigator, or by primary disease category. You can find out if your disorder is under active study and get a listing of current related research projects. If you select a specific study, you will get detailed information about its research protocol, including who may participate and how to join the study. Most studies require a referral from a physician who will submit the person's diagnosis and medical history to the study's principal investigator. The NIH also recruits healthy volunteers for comparison with patient participants. Healthy volunteers are compensated for their time and, sometimes, for the inconvenience of their participation. In some cases, family members are needed to serve as healthy controls for participants in a clinical trial.

The National Cancer Institute (see page 161), although it is part of the NIH, maintains its own listings for up-to-the-minute information on where and how patients can participate in cancer research. The AIDS Clinical Trials Information Service of the National Library of Medicine maintains two databases, AIDSTRIALS and AIDSDRUGS, to provide timely listings of current AIDS-related research trials for both adults and children, plus specific information about the drugs that are currently being tested (see page 148). The databases cover both government-funded and independent research projects.

Major medical centers and universities perform government-backed research and fund research projects of their own. Contact teaching and research hospitals in your area for more information. National associations and support groups for specific diseases are also excellent sources of information about up-to-date research. An Internet search should help you find many research-related sites, including national and international indexes of clinical trials and listings from major research centers across the United States. As with any Internet search, make sure the information you're reading comes from a reliable source.

An alternative therapy you are interested in may be a subject of government research. When you volunteer for an alternative therapy trial that has been approved by the NIH, you will receive the treatment under controlled clinical standards, including careful monitoring for any adverse effects. To check out alternative therapies now being studied under grants from the NIH, contact the National Center for Complementary and Alternative Medicine Clearinghouse (see page 203).

When considering participating in any clinical trial, make sure that all research safeguards are in place, including your right to be fully informed. Ask questions, make sure this is the best choice for you, and always be ready to walk away if you find it necessary.

Doing Your Own Research

You've talked to your physician, the nurse, and maybe a specialist. You've asked questions and read the materials they gave you. How can you find out more? The world is brimming with medical information and health advice—on television, in magazines and newspapers, and on the Internet. The real problem is getting information that is up-to-date, accurate, and reliable.

Where should you go for more in-depth information? First, ask your physician if he or she can recommend scientific journal articles or other professional sources. Check with your local library. A word search on the library's reference computer should net a variety of books and magazine articles. Look for the most recent titles from the most credible sources. Also, megabookstores contain aisles of health-related reading material. If your health questions touch on a popular topic, such as depression, attention-deficit hyperactivity disorder, or vitamin use, you'll find plenty of sources. Bookstore offerings are likely to be more up-to-date than most library listings. However, they also may be more sensational. Scan the shelves of books related to your area of interest, considering an author's credentials and a book's tone and intention. A popular press book may serve as a starting point for more in-depth research.

Search the Internet. The health business is booming on the Web. In fact, health-related sites are getting more "hits" than almost any other kind. Many medical information sites are sponsored by leading medical institutions and highly respected medical companies. Once at a site, you can call up answers to all kinds of healthcare questions. These sites offer plenty of preventive and self-care advice, in-depth information about some diseases, and lists of clinical trials you can join. Be cautious, however. On even some of the best, most reputable sites, the line between editorial content and advertising may be blurred. A list of recommended healthcare centers in your area may actually be a list of institutions that paid to be included on the list. Advice about treatment plans also may be related to sponsorship. Your task will be not so much searching for information as weeding out the inaccurate information. See the Resources section starting on page 141 for useful sites.

National associations and support groups for people with your disorder can be located easily on the Internet. You may find a support group of people who keep in touch with each other and share ideas and problems. By joining a disease-related e-mail list, you can make sure you are constantly updated about new developments in treatment.

Information about drugs and other health products is at your fingertips on the Internet. Type in the name of your prescription medication and you will get plenty of information about it. Sort through it, however, to find out what is relevant and what may be misleading. The information is often provided by pharmaceutical firms or consumer groups. Read everything skeptically.

Finding Reliable Health Information

Q I am often confused by conflicting information I hear in the health reports every day on the evening news. It seems that one study says one thing and the next day another study says something contradicting it. How do I know what to believe?

A In general, the most reliable health information comes from government organizations such as the Centers for Disease Control and Prevention (CDC), major public health organizations such as the American Medical Association, and your doctor. Health studies that make the news vary widely with respect to long-term significance or meaning. For example, if the number of participants in a study was only 10, 20, or even 50 people, the results of the study, however promising, are not likely to be conclusive. Do not allow the results of one study to determine your health and lifestyle choices. Talk to your doctor about what you have heard or read in the media. He or she will help you interpret and understand this information in the context of your own health and lifestyle so that you can make informed decisions. Or if you have access to the Internet, see if you can find more information on a study and doctors' responses to it.

You can even make a cyberspace appointment with an online physician, chat about health concerns, and receive treatment information for a common ailment on the Internet. Sounds simple, but it can be dangerous. You are, in effect, diagnosing yourself by what you choose to tell the doctor or fail to tell him or her. A lengthy chat with a physician online may not uncover a medical problem that a physician could observe easily in a 10-minute office visit. There is no good substitute for a physical examination and an in-person medical evaluation by your doctor. Check the credentials of anyone you chat with online. The physician considering your symptoms may not be a specialist in the area of your particular problem.

You should also approach online pharmacies with caution. Hundreds of pharmacies, some legitimate, some not, have appeared in this uncharted area of cybermedicine. Deaths have occurred from drug interactions caused by improperly prescribed drugs. To avoid problems, use online pharmacies only to fill prescriptions from your own physician. Stay away from Internet pharmacies that don't offer information on how to contact their pharmacists. Be wary of overseas pharmacies because they may sell drugs that are not properly tested or approved for use in the United States.

Resources

The following list of organizations provides a starting point for consumers who are searching for information and resources regarding their health and healthcare. Most of the organizations listed have toll-free telephone numbers, fax numbers, and TDD/TTY numbers for people who are hearing- or speech-impaired. Many groups in this list also have Web sites. You may write, call, fax, or visit a group's Web site for additional information and assistance.

Advocacy

AARP
601 E St., NW
Washington, DC 20049
phone: 800-424-3410
Web site: http://www.aarp.org

AARP (formerly known as the American Association of Retired Persons) is a membership group that provides information, education, advocacy, and community services to meet the needs of people who are age 50 years or older. There are local AARP chapters across the country, and you need not be retired to join. The AARP publishes *Modern Maturity* magazine and the monthly *AARP Bulletin* and offers information on a wide variety of topics that are of interest to older people, including caregiving, long-term care, housing, and financial planning. An AARP membership card entitles you to many different discounts in travel and other purchases.

Asociación Nacional Por Personas Mayores
(National Association for Hispanic Elderly)
1452 W. Temple St., Suite 100
Los Angeles, CA 90026
phone: 213-202-5900
fax: 213-202-5905

Asociación Nacional Por Personas Mayores (ANPPM) is an advocacy group that works to make sure that the needs of older Hispanic people are recognized and that they have access to social service programs. The ANPPM provides training and technical assistance to community groups and professionals in the field of gerontology (the study of aging). The ANPPM conducts market studies and research on aging in the Hispanic community through its National Hispanic Research Center and publishes and distributes Spanish-English information on older Hispanic people and low-income older people through its Hispanic Media Center. The Senior Community Service Employment Program, which is funded by the US Department of Labor and administered by ANPPM, employs low-income people 55 years of age and older in eight states and Puerto Rico. Project Aliento (New Hope) is dedicated to improving access to and broadening the base of agencies and groups that provide services to older Hispanic people and their families. The ANPPM also provides information, referrals, and direct social services and publishes articles, brochures, and audiovisual materials on Social Security, Medicare, health-related topics, and how to start a volunteer group to serve low-income people. Publications are available in both Spanish and English.

B'nai B'rith
1640 Rhode Island Ave., NW
Washington, DC 20036-3278
phone: 202-857-6589
membership services center: 888-388-4BBI (888-388-4224)
fax: 202-857-1099
Web site: http://www.bnaibrith.org

B'nai B'rith, the oldest and largest Jewish service organization in the world, is dedicated to community service, Jewish education, and public advocacy. The B'nai B'rith Center for Senior Housing and Services sponsors and maintains nonsectarian, federally subsidized housing for seniors; conducts continuing education, recreation, and other activities and events; and advocates on behalf of issues of importance to seniors (such as expanded senior housing) in cooperation with the B'nai B'rith Center for Public Policy.

Catholic Charities USA
1731 King St., Suite 200
Alexandria, VA 22314
phone: 703-549-1390
fax: 703-549-1656
Web site: http://www.catholiccharitiesusa.org

Catholic Charities USA is a nationwide social-service organization that provides assistance to people of all ages and backgrounds who are in need. The organization offers a wide range of services for older people, such as counseling, homemaker services, foster family programs, group homes and institutional care, public access programs, caregiver services, and emergency assistance and shelter. Catholic Charities USA also works to advance the rights of older people with regard to employment, housing, and Social Security benefits.

Gray Panthers

733 15th St., NW, Suite 437
Washington, DC 20005
phone: 800-280-5362 or 202-737-6637
fax: 202-737-1160

Gray Panthers is an advocacy group that works toward social change for the benefit of older people and the rest of society in areas such as healthcare, housing, environment, education, and attitudes about aging. Local chapters sponsor public education seminars and organize groups of younger and older people to work together on important social issues. Gray Panthers offers information and referral services for resources for older people. The group also gathers and distributes information on research in gerontology (the study of aging). Members receive *NET-WORK Newsletter*, a bimonthly newsletter. You may call or write to request a list of publications.

National Academy of Elder Law Attorneys, Inc.

1604 N. Country Club Rd.
Tucson, AZ 85716-3102
phone: 520-881-4005
fax: 520-325-7925
Web site: http://www.naela.com

The National Academy of Elder Law Attorneys, Inc., is a nonprofit professional organization that provides information, education, assistance, and networking for lawyers and others who work with older people and their families. The academy can refer you to a lawyer in your area who specializes in handling legal matters that are of particular concern to older people.

National Asian Pacific Center on Aging
Melbourne Tower
1511 3rd Ave., Suite 914
Seattle, WA 98101
phone: 206-624-1221
fax: 206-623-3573
Web site: http://www.napca.org

The National Asian Pacific Center on Aging is a private, nationwide organization dedicated to improving healthcare and social services for older people who are members of the Asian Pacific community in the United States. The center provides assistance to community groups, maintains a national network of service agencies, conducts workshops and training programs for healthcare and social service professionals, and provides information and referrals for family and community support groups. The center also employs older people through its nationwide Seniors' Community Service Employment Program. Publications available include *Asian Pacific Affairs* (published bimonthly) and *The Registry of Services for Asian Pacific Elders*.

National Association of Professional Geriatric Care Managers
1604 N. Country Club Rd.
Tucson, AZ 85716-3102
phone: 520-881-8008
fax: 520-325-7925
Web site: http://www.caremanager.org

The National Association of Professional Geriatric Care Managers is a professional organization dedicated to promoting quality, cost-effective healthcare and human services for older people and their families. The association publishes a nationwide referral directory of professional geriatric care managers that is available for sale.

National Council on the Aging, Inc.
409 3rd St., SW
Washington, DC 20024
phone: 202-479-1200
TDD/TTY phone: 202-479-6674
fax: 202-479-0735
Web site: http://www.ncoa.org

The National Council on the Aging (NCOA) is a private, non-profit organization that serves as a resource for information, technical assistance, training, advocacy, and leadership for service providers and consumers in all aspects of aging. The NCOA publishes a wide range of literature on topics of interest to older people, their families, and healthcare professionals. The NCOA is especially knowledgeable about senior centers, adult day care, long-term care, senior housing, and issues regarding older people who live in rural areas. The NCOA also is home to the National Institute on Adult Daycare.

National Senior Citizens Law Center
Washington, DC office
1101 14th St., NW, Suite 400
Washington, DC 20005
phone: 202-289-6976
fax: 202-289-7224
Los Angeles office
3435 Wilshire Blvd., Suite 2860
Los Angeles, CA 90010-1938
phone: 213-639-0930
fax: 213-639-0934
Web site: http://www.nsclc.org

The National Senior Citizens Law Center (NSCLC) is a public-interest law firm devoted to meeting the legal needs (including legal problems with Social Security, Medicare, Medicaid, age discrimination, pension rights, home healthcare, and nursing facilities) of low-income older people. The NSCLC does not usually handle individual clients but provides information, referral, and consulting services and technical assistance to legal aid offices and attorneys in private practice who serve older, low-income clients. A variety of helpful manuals and reference documents for consumers are available from the NSCLC for a nominal charge. To consult with an NSCLC attorney, write or fax a full description of your legal problem to the office nearest you. You must include your full name, address, and telephone number in all correspondence with the NSCLC. Be sure, also, to include a description (including dates) of any contact you have had with an attorney about your problem.

National Women's Health Network
514 10th St., NW, Suite 400
Washington, DC 20004
phone: 202-347-1140 or 202-628-7814
fax: 202-347-1168
Web site: http://www.womenshealthnetwork.org

The National Women's Health Network (NWHN) is the only national, independent, public-interest membership organization devoted solely to women and health. The NWHN accepts no money from pharmaceutical companies, medical device manufacturers, or tobacco companies. It is an advocate for national health policies that address women's health needs. Members may call or write to get answers to health questions on topics such as hormone replacement, abortion, breast cancer, breast implants, endometriosis, fibroids, ovarian cancer, premenstrual syndrome (PMS), yeast infections, osteoporosis, and menopause. Members get a bimonthly newsletter and reduced rates on network publications.

Clinical Trials

AIDS Clinical Trials Information Service
P.O. Box 6421
Rockville, MD 20849-6421
phone: 800-TRIALS-A (800-874-2572) or 301-517-0459
TDD/TTY phone: 888-480-3739
fax: 301-519-6616
Web site: http://www.actis.org

The AIDS Clinical Trials Information Service (ACTIS) provides quick and easy access to information on federally and privately funded clinical trials for adults and children. ACTIS is sponsored by the US Food and Drug Administration, the National Institute of Allergy and Infectious Diseases, the National Library of Medicine, and the Centers for Disease Control and Prevention.

Office for Human Research Protections
Department of Health and Human Services
6100 Executive Blvd., Suite 3B01, MSC-7507
Rockville, MD 20892-7507
phone: 301-594-2921
fax: 301-402-7065
e-mail: ohrp@osophs.dhhs.gov
Web site: http://ohrp.osophs.dhhs.gov

The Office for Human Research Protections (OHRP) fulfills the responsibilities toward patients that are set forth in the Public Health Service Act. The OHRP ensures that protection regulations for human subjects are appropriately and effectively applied. It also conducts inquiries and investigations into alleged noncompliance with US Department of Health and Human Services regulations and recommends remedial or corrective action.

Warren Grant Magnuson Clinical Center
National Institutes of Health
6100 Executive Blvd., Room 3C01
Bethesda, MD 20892-4754
To participate in clinical research:
phone: 800-411-1222
fax: 301-480-9793
e-mail: prpl@mail.cc.nih.gov
For general information:
phone: 301-496-2563
fax: 301-402-2984
Web site: http://www.cc.nih.gov

The clinical center of the National Institutes of Health (NIH) is a federally funded biomedical research facility and is the research hospital for the NIH. It supports clinical investigations conducted by the institutes and opportunities for physicians and patients to participate in cutting-edge research and scientific advances. The clinical center is specially designed to bring patient-care facilities in proximity to research laboratories. At the patient recruitment and referral center, staff members assist patients, their families, and physicians by providing information about participating in research at the clinical center. Although referral by a medical practitioner is preferable, trained nurses will answer questions and send information about the program and the admission process to patients under some circumstances. A preliminary screening interview may be conducted. Staff also will refer physicians to a contact person who can provide more details about the studies and the criteria for patient referral.

Diseases and Conditions

Alzheimer's Association
919 N. Michigan Ave., Suite 1100
Chicago, IL 60611-1676
phone: 800-272-3900 or 312-335-8700
fax: 312-335-1110
Web site: http://www.alz.org

The Alzheimer's Association sponsors advocacy, research, and education programs and offers care and support services through a network of local chapters. The association also sponsors various national conferences (such as the National Education Conference), events (such as Memory Walk, a national fundraiser), and programs (such as Safe Return, a nationwide identification program for locating lost or disoriented people and reuniting them with their families). The Alzheimer's Association publishes *Advances*, a quarterly newsletter for families affected by the disease, and *Research & Practice*, a newsletter for healthcare professionals. The association's Benjamin B. Green–Field Library and Resource Center has a wide range of informational materials (such as books, journals, videos, audiocassettes, and CD-ROMs) available for use on site or through interlibrary loan. Your local chapter can provide information, support, referrals, and other types of assistance.

Alzheimer's Disease Education and Referral Center
P.O. Box 8250
Silver Springs, MD 20907-8250
phone: 800-438-4380
fax: 301-495-3334
Web site: http://www.alzheimers.org

The Alzheimer's Disease Education and Referral Center (ADEAR Center) is a service of the National Institute on Aging

(NIA), which is part of the National Institutes of Health. The ADEAR Center answers questions about Alzheimer's disease, including questions about research findings and new treatments. The center also offers free publications and can provide information on and referrals to diagnosis and treatment centers, drug trials, and support groups.

American Academy of Dermatology
930 N. Meacham Rd.
Schaumburg, IL 60173
phone: 847-330-0230 or 888-462-DERM (888-462-3376)
Web site: http://www.aad.org

The American Academy of Dermatology (AAD) is the largest of all dermatology associations and is a highly influential one. Although its principal objective is continuing medical education in dermatology for physicians, the academy plays a major role in formulating socioeconomic policies. AAD also supports enhanced patient care and public interest in dermatology-related issues. Informational brochures on more than 35 skin, hair, and nail conditions are available. Through its Web site, the general public can find a dermatologist by area code, zip code, last name, city, state, or country and biographical profile.

American Cancer Society
1599 Clifton Rd., NE
Atlanta, GA 30329-4251
info-line phone: 800-ACS-2345 (800-227-2345)
national office phone: 404-320-3333
fax: 512-927-5791
Web site: http://www.cancer.org

The American Cancer Society provides a wide range of services to people with cancer, their families and caregivers, and the general public. Both emotional and practical assistance are available. The American Cancer Society offers a number of educational programs and support groups (for example, Reach to Recovery is a visitation program for women with breast cancer, and Man to Man is a support program for men with prostate cancer). The American Cancer Society also offers free pamphlets and brochures, transportation to and from medical treatments, lodging assistance, and children's camps for children who have or have had cancer. Another service of the American Cancer Society is the *TLC Catalogue*, which offers medical information and special products for women recently diagnosed with breast cancer, breast cancer survivors, and women with treatment-related hair loss.

American College of Cardiology

Heart House
9111 Old Georgetown Rd.
Bethesda, MD 20814-1699
phone: 800-253-4636 or 301-897-5400
fax: 301-897-9745
Web site: http://www.acc.org

The American College of Cardiology (ACC) is an international professional society of cardiovascular physicians and scientists. Members have special knowledge and experience in treating heart disorders. The college offers patient education materials and referrals to board-certified cardiologists.

American College of Gastroenterology

4900B S. 31st St.
Arlington, VA 22206-1656
phone: 703-820-7400
fax: 703-931-4520
Web site: http://www.acg.gi.org

The American College of Gastroenterology (ACG) advances

the study and medical treatment of disorders of the digestive, or gastrointestinal, tract. ACG is guided by its commitment to meeting the needs of clinical gastroenterologists. The college's goals are to advance knowledge of, and education in, gastrointestinal disease; represent the interests of gastroenterologists; ensure quality of patient care; and promote patient education on gastrointestinal conditions and digestive health. Topics such as "Understanding Your Gastrointestinal Tract," "What Everyone Should Know About Colon Cancer," "Understanding GERD," and "Digestive Health Tips" are further explored on ACG's extensive Web site. You also can find an ACG member in your state with the GI Physician Locator.

American Diabetes Association
1701 N. Beauregard St.
Alexandria, VA 22314
phone: 800-DIABETES (800-342-2383) or 703-549-1500
Web site: http://www.diabetes.org

The American Diabetes Association (ADA) fights diabetes through education and research. Local chapters provide a wide range of services, including diabetes education classes, year-round youth programs, counseling and support groups, advocacy services, and referral services. The ADA sponsors a special African American Program designed to increase diabetes awareness among African Americans. The program offers community-based activities such as Diabetes Sunday, Get Up and Move, and Healthy Eating, and publishes a newsletter, *In Touch*. For people with diabetes, the ADA publishes *Diabetes Forecast*, a health and wellness magazine, and *Diabetes Advisor*, a bimonthly newsletter with easy-to-understand information on self-care for people who are just learning to live with diabetes. The ADA also publishes books, brochures, and pamphlets on every aspect of living with diabetes and a comprehensive collection of cookbooks, meal-planning guides, and food-exchange lists. You may purchase ADA books at your local bookstore or directly from the ADA. Call the ADA's toll-free information and referral line or write to customer service at the address above to request a free diabetes information packet.

American Heart Association
National Center
7272 Greenville Ave.
Dallas, TX 75231-4596
phone: 800-AHA-USA1 (800-242-8721) or 214-373-6300
Web site: http://www.americanheart.org

The American Heart Association (AHA) is a nonprofit, volunteer agency that strives to reduce death and disability caused by cardiovascular disease, such as heart disease and stroke, through education, advocacy, and research. The AHA publishes informational materials on all aspects of cardiovascular disease; its books are widely available in bookstores. The AHA Web site offers helpful information on topics such as warning signs, risk assessment, prevention, treatment, and recovery, and provides links to other online sources of useful information. The association's Web site also has an easy-to-use A–Z reference guide to heart disease and stroke.

American Stroke Association
National Center
7272 Greenville Ave.
Dallas, TX 75231-4596
phone: 888-4-STROKE (888-478-7653)
Stroke Connection phone: 800-553-6321
Web site: http://www.strokeassociation.org

The American Stroke Association is a division of the American Heart Association that provides nationwide information and referrals for people who have had strokes, their families and caregivers, and the general public. The people who handle calls at the American Stroke Association are dedicated to serving stroke survivors and their families and educating the general public about stroke. You can call for answers to specific questions about stroke or referrals to support groups, or you can ask to talk to someone who has had experiences similar to yours. *Stroke Connection* magazine is written by stroke survivors and caregivers for stroke survivors and their families and caregivers. The magazine contains helpful information about prevention, early treatment, and rehabilitation and offers support, hope, and encouragement to stroke survivors and their families. *Stroke Connection* magazine is available by subscription or online.

Arthritis Foundation
1330 W. Peachtree St.
Atlanta, GA 30309
phone: 800-283-7800 or 404-872-7100
Web site: http://www.arthritis.org

The Arthritis Foundation is a nonprofit volunteer organization dedicated to improving the quality of life for people with arthritis. The Arthritis Foundation supports research and offers continuing education programs and publications for healthcare professionals. Local chapters provide information and referral services for people with arthritis and their families. They also offer educational programs including self-help courses, exercise programs, and support groups. The Arthritis Foundation has a large selection of helpful brochures, booklets, videos, and other resources available free or for a modest charge. The foundation also publishes a bimonthly consumer magazine for members.

Asthma and Allergy Foundation of America
1233 20th St., NW, Suite 402
Washington, DC 20036

phone: 800-7-ASTHMA (800-727-8462) or 202-466-7643
fax: 202-466-8940
Web site: http://www.aafa.org

The Asthma and Allergy Foundation of America (AAFA) is a nonprofit organization that works to control and to find a cure for asthma and allergic diseases. The AAFA serves the public through research, educational programs for patients and the public, direct individual and family support through local chapters and educational support groups, public awareness campaigns, and advocacy. The AAFA produces several subscription newsletters, including *The Asthma and Allergy Advance*, a bimonthly patient education newsletter; *HealthLines SAY*, a bimonthly newsletter written by and for adolescents living with asthma and allergies; and *Asthma & Allergy Exchange*, a quarterly newsletter for healthcare professionals. The AAFA offers a number of asthma education programs and a variety of educational materials such as books, games, and videos that can be ordered from the foundation at a discount to members. Contact AAFA for additional information and to request a list of available educational materials.

Brain Injury Association, Inc.
105 N. Alfred St.
Alexandria, VA 22314
phone: 703-236-6000
family helpline: 800-444-6443
fax: 703-236-6001
Web site: http://www.biausa.org

The Brain Injury Association (BIA) helps people locate and develop community-based resources, supports medical research and legislation, and sponsors conferences and meetings. The BIA offers consumers helpful information on topics such as prevention, treatment, rehabilitation, and living with a brain injury. The BIA also sponsors interactive multimedia brain injury resource centers, which provide easy-to-understand information for families and more complex information for healthcare professionals. The information includes answers to questions about brain injury, a glossary of medical and technical terms, and descriptions of professionals who deal with brain injury and the services they offer. Also provided are interviews with people who have a brain injury, family members, and professionals at various stages of recovery and a list of educational and informational materials that are available for purchase.

Cancer Information Service
phone: 800-4-CANCER (800-422-6237)
TDD/TTY phone: 800-332-8615
Web site: http://cis.nci.nih.gov

The Cancer Information Service (CIS) is supported by the National Cancer Institute, the federal agency that coordinates the government's cancer research programs. The CIS answers questions about cancer and cancer-related issues and offers free literature and other resources. The CIS also provides information on the latest clinical studies and experimental treatment programs.

HeartInfo
Web site: http://www.heartinfo.org

HeartInfo is an independent, educational Web site dedicated to providing information and services to people with a cardiovascular disorder. The site is geared toward consumers and is managed by Daniel James Rader, MD, director of the Lipid Referral Center and the Cardiovascular Risk Intervention Program at the University of Pennsylvania Health System. You will find material about heart disease, the latest news on treatment options, and information on available products and services.

Heart Information Service
Texas Heart Institute
P.O. Box 20345
Houston, TX 77225-0345
phone: 800-292-2221 or 713-794-6536
fax: 713-794-3714
Web site: http://www.tmc.edu/thi

The Heart Information Service, a program of the Texas Heart Institute, is a national hot line that answers questions from the general public regarding the diagnosis, treatment, and prevention of cardiovascular disease.

International Hearing Society
16880 Middlebelt Rd., Suite 4
Livonia, MI 48154
phone: 734-522-7200
Hearing Aid Helpline phone: 800-521-5247, ext. 333
fax: 734-522-0200
Web site: http://www.hearingihs.org

The International Hearing Society (IHS) is a professional organization that sets professional standards and offers continuing education programs for hearing aid specialists. The Hearing Aid Helpline answers questions about hearing aids and hearing loss, deals with consumer complaints about hearing aids, and provides referrals to qualified hearing aid specialists. The helpline operates between 10:00 A.M. and 4:00 P.M., Eastern Time, Monday through Friday. The IHS publishes the *Directory of National Hearing Aid Society Members*. Various other publications that deal with specific questions about hearing aids and hearing loss are available to consumers.

International Tremor Foundation
7046 W. 105th St.

Overland Park, KS 66212-1803
phone: 913-341-3880
fax: 913-341-1296
Web site: http://www.essentialtremor.org

The International Tremor Foundation is a nonprofit membership organization that provides information and referral services
for people who have tremor disorders and their families. The
foundation supports research on tremor disorders and publishes
a quarterly newsletter for its members. The foundation also
offers a variety of publications on tremor disorders.

**National Arthritis and Musculoskeletal and Skin Diseases
Information Clearinghouse**
1 AMS Cir.
Bethesda, MD 20892-3675
phone: 301-495-4484
TDD/TTY phone: 301-565-2966
fax: 301-718-6366
NIAMS Fast Fax System: 301-881-2731
Web site: http://www.nih.gov/niams

The National Arthritis and Musculoskeletal and Skin Diseases
Information Clearinghouse is part of the National Institute of
Arthritis and Musculoskeletal and Skin Diseases (NIAMS). The
NIAMS is part of the National Institutes of Health, the US
government's principal biomedical research agency. The
NIAMS supports and conducts clinical research and provides
up-to-date information for use by the public and healthcare
professionals via fact sheets, brochures, health statistics, reports,
and scientific research databases and other biomedical resources
on the Internet. The NIAMS can answer your questions about
issues and products related to arthritis and diseases of the musculoskeletal system and skin.

National Association for Continence
P.O. Box 8310
Spartanburg, SC 29305-8310
phone: 800-BLADDER (800-252-3337) or 864-579-7900
fax: 864-579-7902
Web site: http://www.nafc.org

The National Association for Continence (NAFC) is a nonprofit membership organization that works to improve the quality of life for people with incontinence. The NAFC conducts education, advocacy, service, and support programs and focuses on causes, prevention, diagnosis, treatment, and management alternatives. The NAFC publishes *Quality Care*, a quarterly newsletter, and *The Resource Guide—Products and Services for Incontinence*, a directory of products and manufacturers. The NAFC also provides helpful information (such as pamphlets, videos, and books) on dealing with urinary incontinence and fecal incontinence for both consumers and healthcare professionals.

National Association of the Deaf
814 Thayer Ave.
Silver Springs, MD 20910-4500
phone: 301-587-1788
TDD/TTY phone: 301-587-1789
fax: 301-587-1791
Web site: http://www.nad.org

The National Association of the Deaf (NAD) is a nonprofit advocacy organization that serves the needs of people who are deaf or hearing-impaired. The association answers questions from the general public and supports a variety of programs, including Youth Leadership Camp, Junior NAD, Interpreter and Sign Language Interpreter certification, and the Legal Defense Fund. The NAD also offers a variety of books and other informative publications about hearing loss and deafness.

National Cancer Institute
Office of Communications
31 Center Dr., MSC-2580
Bethesda, MD 20892-2580
phone: 800-4-CANCER (800-422-6237)
public inquiries office phone: 301-435-3848
Web site: http://www.nci.nih.gov

The National Cancer Institute (NCI) can help locate answers to cancer-related questions but cannot answer personal medical questions or provide consultations. The NCI also maintains listings of up-to-the-minute information on where and how patients can participate in cancer trials for cancer research. Go to the NCI Web site to find answers to inquiries about the institute's activities.

National Center for HIV, STD, and TB Prevention
1600 Clifton Rd., NE
Atlanta, GA 30333
phone: 404-639-3311
national STD hot line: 800-227-8922
national AIDS hot lines (24 hours a day, 7 days a week):
English: 800-342-AIDS (800-342-2437)
Spanish: 800-344-SIDA (800-344-7432)
TDD/TTY phone: 800-243-7889
fax: 888-CDC-FAXX (888-232-3299)
e-mail: hivmail@cdc.gov
Web site: http://www.cdc.gov/hiv/dhap.htm

The National Center for HIV, STD, and TB Prevention is part of the Centers for Disease Control and Prevention. The center provides general information on HIV, AIDS, STDs, and tuberculosis. You can find journal articles about these diseases, along with the latest on prevention, treatment, laboratory research, funding, vaccines, and testing. Consult the Web site for frequently asked questions and to find information on brochures, fact sheets, statistics, conferences, and publications. The confidential hot lines will put you in touch with a person trained to answer questions. He or she also will tell you where to get clinical services and other help.

National Center for Vision and Aging
The Lighthouse International
111 E. 59th St., 11th floor
New York, NY 10022-1202
Information and Resource Service phone: 800-829-0500
TDD/TTY phone: 212-821-9713
New York area phone: 212-821-9200
fax: 212-821-9705
Web site: http://www.lighthouse.org

The National Center for Vision and Aging (NCVA), a division of The Lighthouse, Inc., assists older people who have, or who are at risk of developing, impaired vision. The NCVA conducts research on aging-related vision impairment and provides a continuing education program for professionals. The NCVA Information and Resource Service offers consumers helpful information on a variety of topics, including eye diseases and conditions and assistive devices, and can refer callers to vision rehabilitation agencies, low-vision centers, and support groups. The NCVA also produces a wide variety of educational materials for consumers. The *Lighthouse Consumer Catalog* offers a number of useful products for people who have impaired vision.

National Clearinghouse for Alcohol and Drug Information
P.O. Box 2345
Rockville, MD 20847-2345
phone: 800-729-6686
TDD/TTY phone: 800-487-4889

fax: 301-468-6433

Web site: http://www.health.org

The National Clearinghouse for Alcohol and Drug Information is the largest resource for current information and materials about substance abuse (including alcohol and tobacco). Prevention Online (PREVLINE), a service provided by the clearinghouse, provides information about specific drugs.

National Diabetes Information Clearinghouse
1 Information Way
Bethesda, MD 20892-3560
phone: 301-654-3327
fax: 301-907-8906
Web site: http://www.niddk.nih.gov

The National Diabetes Information Clearinghouse (NDIC) is an information and referral service of the National Institute of Diabetes and Digestive and Kidney Diseases (see page 165). The NDIC is designed to increase knowledge and understanding about diabetes among people with diabetes, their families, healthcare professionals, and the general public. The NDIC responds to written requests for information and offers a variety of fact sheets, brochures, pamphlets, booklets, reports, and reprints on diabetes to consumers. The NDIC publishes a quarterly newsletter, *Diabetes Dateline*, and *The Diabetes Dictionary*, an illustrated glossary of more than 350 diabetes-related terms. Consumers may search for additional information on diabetes on the Combined Health Information Database, which is accessible through the NDIC Web site.

National Digestive Diseases Information Clearinghouse
2 Information Way
Bethesda, MD 20892-3570
phone: 301-654-3810

fax: 301-907-8906

Web site: http://www.niddk.nih.gov

The National Digestive Diseases Information Clearinghouse (NDDIC) is an information and referral service of the National Institute of Diabetes and Digestive and Kidney Diseases (see page 165). The NDDIC is designed to increase knowledge and understanding about digestive diseases—for example, pancreatitis, inflammatory bowel disease, hepatitis, ulcers, and gallstones—among people with digestive diseases, their families, healthcare professionals, and the general public. The NDDIC responds to written requests for information and offers a variety of fact sheets, brochures, pamphlets, booklets, reports, and reprints on digestive diseases to consumers. The NDDIC publishes a newsletter, *DD Notes*, that features news and information about digestive diseases. Consumers may search for additional information on digestive diseases on the Combined Health Information Database, which is accessible through the NDDIC Web site.

National Heart, Lung, and Blood Institute Information Center
P.O. Box 30105
Bethesda, MD 20824-0105
phone: 301-592-8573
recorded wellness information: 800-575-WELL
   (800-575-9355)
fax: 301-592-8563
Web site: http://www.nhlbi.nih.gov

The National Heart, Lung, and Blood Institute (NHLBI) plans, conducts, and supports a program of research and education in diseases of the heart, lungs, blood, and blood vessels; blood resources; and sleep disorders. The NHLBI Information

Center seeks to improve public health by translating the results of medical research into practical consumer information and advice. The information center serves as a clearinghouse for brochures, audiovisual materials, cookbooks, and many more helpful materials. The Web site contains a section on "studies seeking patients" for those interested in participating in research.

National Institute of Diabetes and Digestive and Kidney Diseases

31 Center Dr., Building 31, Room 9A-04, MSC-2560
Bethesda, MD 20892-2560
phone: 301-496-3583
fax: 301-496-7422
Web site: http://www.niddk.nih.gov

The National Institute of Diabetes and Digestive and Kidney Diseases (NIDDK) is part of the National Institutes of Health, the US government's principal biomedical research agency. The NIDDK conducts research and administers the National Diabetes Education Program, the National Diabetes Information Clearinghouse, the National Digestive Diseases Information Clearinghouse, the National Kidney and Urologic Diseases Information Clearinghouse, and the Weight-Control Information Network. The NIDDK publishes a wide variety of free fact sheets, brochures, and pamphlets for consumers on topics such as diabetes, digestive diseases, kidney and urologic diseases, weight control, and nutrition.

National Institute of Neurologic Disorders and Stroke

Office of Communications and Public Liaison
31 Center Dr., Building 31, Room 8A-18, MSC-2540
Bethesda, MD 20892-2540
phone: 301-496-5751

fax: 301-402-2186

Web site: http://www.ninds.nih.gov

The National Institute of Neurologic Disorders and Stroke conducts and supports research on the causes, prevention, diagnosis, and treatment of stroke and other disorders of the brain and nervous system. Consumer-oriented publications on a variety of topics are available.

National Institutes of Health Office of Rare Diseases
31 Center Dr., Building 31, Room 1B-19, MSC-2084
Bethesda, MD 20892-2082
phone: 301-402-4336
fax: 301-402-0420
Web site: http://rarediseases.info.nih.gov/ord

The Office of Rare Diseases of the National Institutes of Health provides information on more than 6,000 rare diseases and conditions. You can find causes, treatments, and definitions of technical language, along with a list of publications on the Web site. There also are progress reports on rare-disease research and clinical trials, a calendar of events, and links to patient support groups and sources that are useful to research investigators. There are also extensive data on genetic testing, genetic counselors, and counseling centers. Lodging and patient travel updates to research and treatment sites also are available. If your physician has mentioned that a particular research project might be helpful in treating you or a member of your family, this Web site is a good place to look for more information on the study.

National Kidney and Urologic Diseases Information Clearinghouse
3 Information Way
Bethesda, MD 20892-3570
phone: 301-654-4415

fax: 301-907-8906

Web site: http://www.niddk.nih.gov

The National Kidney and Urologic Diseases Information Clearinghouse (NKUDIC) is an information and referral service of the National Institute of Diabetes and Digestive and Kidney Diseases (see page 165). The NKUDIC is designed to increase knowledge and understanding about kidney and urologic diseases—including end-stage renal disease, urinary stone disease, urinary incontinence, benign prostatic hyperplasia, interstitial cystitis, urinary tract infection, and polycystic kidney disease—among people who have such diseases, their families, healthcare professionals, and the general public. The NKUDIC responds to written requests for information and offers a variety of fact sheets, brochures, pamphlets, booklets, reports, and reprints on kidney and urologic diseases to consumers. The NKUDIC publishes a newsletter, *KU Notes*. Consumers may search for additional information on diabetes and urologic diseases on the Combined Health Information Database, which is accessible through the NKUDIC Web site.

National Kidney Foundation
30 E. 33rd St., Suite 1100
New York, NY 10016
phone: 800-622-9010 or 212-889-2210
fax: 212-689-9261
Web site: http://www.kidney.org

The National Kidney Foundation publishes pamphlets on kidney disease and offers health screening, counseling, referrals, transportation, and other programs for people with kidney disease.

National Osteoporosis Foundation
1232 22nd St., NW
Washington, DC 20037-1292

phone: 202-223-2226
fax: 202-223-2237
Web site: http://www.nof.org

The National Osteoporosis Foundation (NOF) is a voluntary organization that works to increase awareness and knowledge of osteoporosis among people who have or who are at risk of developing this condition, their families, healthcare professionals, and the general public. The NOF supports osteoporosis research and works to increase federal funding for such research and publishes a variety of materials for consumers, including *Osteoporosis: A Woman's Guide* and *An Older Person's Guide to Osteoporosis.* The NOF also publishes a quarterly newsletter and provides referrals to local osteoporosis support groups.

National Parkinson Foundation, Inc.
Bob Hope Parkinson Research Center
1501 N.W. 9th Ave.
Miami, FL 33136-1494
phone: 800-327-4545 or 305-547-6666
fax: 305-243-4403
Web site: http://www.parkinson.org

The National Parkinson Foundation is dedicated to finding the cause and cure for Parkinson's disease and related disorders through research. The foundation works to educate healthcare professionals, patients, families, caregivers, and the general public about Parkinson's disease. The foundation distributes a wide variety of free informational literature and sponsors seminars around the United States. The National Parkinson Foundation also sponsors support groups for people with Parkinson's disease and their families and caregivers and encourages formation of new support groups by providing technical assistance and all necessary informational materials. The foundation also provides complete diagnostic services along with physical, occupational, and speech therapies. All patients are treated regardless of their ability to pay. You can request materials, physician referrals, and general information at the toll-free number.

National Stroke Association
9707 E. Easter Lane
Englewood, CO 80112-3747
phone: 800-STROKES (800-787-6537) or 303-649-9299
fax: 303-649-1328
Web site: http://www.stroke.org

The National Stroke Association is a nonprofit volunteer organization dedicated to stroke education and research. The association provides information, referrals, and guidance on forming support groups for people who have had strokes and their families and caregivers. The association also serves as a clearinghouse for information on prevention, detection, and treatment of stroke and offers information on aftercare centers and rehabilitation.

Osteoporosis and Related Bone Diseases Resource Center
1232 22nd St., NW
Washington, DC 20037-1292
phone: 800-624-BONE (800-624-2663) or 202-223-0344
TDD/TTY phone: 202-466-4315
fax: 202-293-2356
Web site: http://www.osteo.org

The Osteoporosis and Related Bone Diseases Resource Center is dedicated to prevention, early detection, and treatment, along with developing coping strategies. The center provides information on and access to other resources to patients, healthcare professionals, and the general public.

Parkinson's Disease Foundation, Inc.

710 W. 168th St.

New York, NY 10032-9982

phone: 800-457-6676

fax: 212-923-4778

Web site: http://www.pdf.org

The Parkinson's Disease Foundation is a nonprofit organization that provides a variety of services to people who have Parkinson's disease and their families, including educational materials, educational programs, a quarterly newsletter, and physician referrals. The foundation supports neurological research and also offers a variety of helpful publications, such as *One Step at a Time* and *The Exercise Program*, to consumers.

United Ostomy Association, Inc.

19772 MacArthur Blvd., Suite 200

Irvine, CA 92612-2405

phone: 800-826-0826

Web site: http://www.uoa.org

United Ostomy Association, Inc. (UOA) is a volunteer-based organization with local chapters throughout the United States dedicated to assisting people who have had or will have intestinal or urinary diversions. The UOA provides preoperative and postoperative visits and support; ostomy and alternative procedures publications; a quarterly magazine; advocacy activities; national, state, and regional conferences; and liaison to other healthcare organizations.

Y-ME National Breast Cancer Organization

212 W. Van Buren St., 5th floor

Chicago, IL 60607-3908

National Breast Cancer hot lines (24 hours a day, 7 days a week):

English: 800-221-2141
Spanish: 800-986-9505
Web site: http://www.y-me.org

Y-ME National Breast Cancer Organization is committed to serving women with breast cancer and their families and friends. Y-ME offers national hot lines, a Web site, and nationwide referrals to mammogram facilities, comprehensive breast centers, and treatment and research hospitals. Y-ME provides support programs, monthly educational and support meetings, public education seminars, special programs on breast health awareness for high school senior girls, and in-service workshops for healthcare professionals. Y-ME also works at the state and federal levels for increased breast cancer research funding, access to quality treatment for all women, and nondiscriminatory legislation. A network of local chapters and support groups operates under the Y-ME name. Y-ME publications include a bimonthly newsletter, *Hotline;* a Spanish-English newsletter, *Noticias Latinas;* and a variety of booklets about breast health and breast cancer. Most information is available in both English and Spanish. Contact the Y-ME National Breast Cancer hot lines for further information and assistance.

General Health Information

American Academy of Pediatrics
141 Northwest Point Blvd.
Elk Grove Village, IL 60007-1098
phone: 847-228-5005
fax: 847-228-5097
Web site: http://www.aap.org

The American Academy of Pediatrics (AAP) is a professional organization dedicated to the health, safety, and well-being of infants, children, and young adults. The AAP publishes books, brochures, and much more on child and adolescent health topics for healthcare professionals and for the general public.

American College of Obstetricians and Gynecologists
409 12th St., SW
P.O. Box 96920
Washington, DC 20090-6920
phone: 202-863-2518
fax: 202-484-1595
Web site: http://www.acog.org

The American College of Obstetricians and Gynecologists (ACOG) is a nonprofit volunteer organization made up of the nation's leading group of professionals providing healthcare for women. The college serves as an advocate for quality healthcare for women, maintains high standards for clinical practice and continuing education, promotes patient education and understanding of medical care, and increases awareness of the changing issues of women's healthcare in both its members and the public. You can obtain patient education pamphlets on subjects such as progestin, D&C, menopause, and gestational diabetes.

American Dietetic Association
216 W. Jackson Blvd., 7th floor
Chicago, IL 60606-6995
phone: 800-366-1655 or 312-899-0040
Web site: http://www.eatright.org

The American Dietetic Association (ADA) promotes the science of nutrition and public education about food, nutrition, and health. You can talk to a registered dietitian or listen to informative recorded messages about nutrition and health by calling the ADA's toll-free number. The ADA also publishes informational materials on a wide variety of nutrition-related topics.

American Geriatrics Society

Empire State Building
350 5th Ave., Suite 801
New York, NY 10118
phone: 212-308-1414
fax: 212-832-8646
Web site: http://www.americangeriatrics.org

The American Geriatrics Society (AGS) is an organization dedicated to improving the health and well-being of older adults and has been influential in affecting healthcare for older adults. The society has an active membership of more than 6,000 physicians, nurses, researchers, educators, pharmacists, physician's assistants, social workers, physical therapists, and healthcare administrators. Anyone with an interest in geriatric healthcare is welcome to join. The AGS ensures the provision of quality healthcare for older adults by developing, implementing, and supporting programs in patient care, research, professional education, and public education and policy.

American Medical Association

515 N. State St.
Chicago, IL 60610
phone: 312-464-5000
Web site: http://www.ama-assn.org

The American Medical Association (AMA) is the largest physician organization in the United States. The AMA serves physicians and their patients by promoting ethical, educational, and clinical standards for the medical profession. The AMA publishes some health information and medical news for consumers and physicians on its own but also is a member organization of Medem (see page 183). Medem is a medical information Web site that provides health-related information from member professional medical societies. If you need a physician, you can access information by medical specialty or by doctor's name under Physician Select: The Doctor Finder on the AMA Web site. Referrals to licensed physicians throughout the United States and its possessions are provided by county medical societies. All physician data have been verified for accuracy and authenticated and can be searched by specialty.

Canadian Medical Association
1867 Alta Vista Dr.
Ottawa, Ontario, Canada K1G 3Y6
phone: 613-731-9331
Web site: http://www.cma.ca

The Canadian Medical Association is a valuable source of medical information and resources. Although this Web site contains information mainly for physicians, it includes book reviews and summaries of recent articles published in the *Canadian Medical Association Journal*. The group's Web site offers information in English and French and contains a search engine that will help you locate links to a wide variety of medical topics.

National Health Information Center
P.O. Box 1133
Washington, DC 20013-1133
phone: 800-336-4797 or 301-565-4167
fax: 301-984-4256 or 301-468-1204
Web site: http://nhic-nt.health.org

The National Health Information Center (NHIC) is a clearinghouse that can help you locate specific health organizations and provide information on the resources and services they offer. Contact the NHIC if you do not know which organization to contact for specific health-related information; you will be directed to the appropriate group.

National Medical Association
1012 10th St., NW
Washington, DC 20001
phone: 202-347-1895
fax: 202-347-0722
Web site: http://www.nmanet.org

The National Medical Association (NMA) is the collective voice of African American physicians and a leading force for parity and justice in medicine and the elimination of disparities in health. Consumers can visit Your Health on the NMA Web site to access up-to-date information on health issues such as breast cancer, glaucoma, AIDS, and asthma; to take action on legislative alerts; and to review the NMA calendar of events to find out about health-related events in their area.

Women's Health Initiative
Rockledge Center
6705 Rockledge Dr., Suite 300
Bethesda, MD 20892-7966
phone: 301-402-2900
Web site: http://www.nhlbi.nih.gov/whi/index.html

The Women's Health Initiative is a 15-year research program designed to study the major causes of death and disability in women and to reduce coronary heart disease, breast and colon cancer, and osteoporosis in postmenopausal women.

Government Agencies

Consumer Product Safety Commission
Washington, DC 20207-0001
English/Spanish phone: 800-638-2772
TDD/TTY phone: 800-638-8270
Web site: http://www.cpsc.gov

The Consumer Product Safety Commission (CPSC) is an independent federal regulatory agency that develops and sets mandatory safety standards for manufacturers, educates the public about product safety, conducts research, and issues and enforces bans and recalls. The agency's purpose is to protect the public against unreasonable risks of injury and death associated with consumer products. The CPSC has jurisdiction over about 15,000 types of consumer products and operates the Injury Information Clearinghouse, which collects information about consumer product-related injuries. The agency also offers a variety of free publications, such as *Home Safety Checklist for Older Consumers* and *Fire Safety Checklist for Older Consumers*. You may write to request a free copy of the CPSC publication list. You may call for information on a specific product or to report an unsafe consumer product or a product-related injury or death.

Eldercare Locator
phone: 800-677-1116

Eldercare Locator, a nationwide directory service established by the National Association of Area Agencies on Aging, provides state and local information and referrals for older people and their caregivers. For example, information and referrals are available for Alzheimer's disease hot lines, adult day-care services, nursing facility ombudsmen, home healthcare complaints, legal assistance, and elder abuse and protective services. Eldercare Locator answers calls Monday through Friday between 9:00 A.M. and 11:00 P.M., Eastern time. After hours, voice mail will record your name and telephone number, and an information specialist will return your call the next business day.

Equal Employment Opportunity Commission
1801 L St., NW
Washington, DC 20507

phone: 800-669-4000
TDD/TTY phone: 800-669-6820
Web site: http://www.eeoc.gov

The Equal Employment Opportunity Commission (EEOC) provides assistance in dealing with discrimination in the workplace, including discrimination based on age, gender, race, color, religion, national origin, or disability.

Food and Drug Administration
5600 Fishers Lane
Rockville, MD 20857-0001
phone: 888-463-6332
fax: 301-443-9767
Web site: http://www.fda.gov

The Food and Drug Administration (FDA) is the federal government's consumer protection agency. The FDA can answer your questions about foods, food supplements, drugs, cosmetics, and medical devices—and how they are regulated.

Health Canada
A.L. 0904A
Ottawa, Ontario, Canada K1A OK9
phone: 613-957-2991
fax: 613-941-5366
Web site: http://www.hc-sc.gc.ca

Health Canada is the federal department that is responsible for helping Canadian citizens maintain their health. The department promotes disease prevention and healthy living. You can search Health Canada's medical database for helpful information on a variety of health-related topics.

National Institute on Adult Daycare
See National Council on the Aging, Inc., page 146.

National Institute on Aging Information Center
P.O. Box 8057
Gaithersburg, MD 20898-8057
phone: 800-222-2225
TDD/TTY phone: 800-222-4225
fax: 301-589-3014
Web sites: http://www.nih.gov/nia and
  http://www.aoa.dhhs.gov

The National Institute on Aging (NIA) is one of the National Institutes of Health, which is the principal biomedical research agency of the US government. The NIA promotes healthy aging by conducting and supporting biomedical, social, and behavioral research and public education. The NIA offers a wide variety of informative free brochures and fact sheets called *Age Pages* on topics of interest to older people, including diseases, disorders, and conditions; health promotion and disease prevention; medical care; medications and immunizations; exercise; nutrition; planning for later years; and safety.

National Institutes of Health
9000 Rockville Pike
Bethesda, MD 20892
phone: 301-496-4000
Web site: http://www.nih.gov

The National Institutes of Health (NIH) is one of eight health agencies that is part of the US Department of Health and Human Services. It is a government agency dedicated to helping prevent, detect, diagnose, and treat disease and disability. It is made up of 25 separate institutes and centers, some of which are noted elsewhere in this resource section.

National Library of Medicine
8600 Rockville Pike

Bethesda, MD 20894
phone: 888-FIND-NLM (888-346-3656)
local and international phone: 301-594-5983
Web site: http://www.nlm.nih.gov
Internet Grateful Med Web site: http://igm.nlm.nih.gov
PubMed Web site: http://www.ncbi.nlm.nih.gov/PubMed

The National Library of Medicine (NLM) is the world's largest medical library and a gold mine of solid medical information of all sorts. By using the NLM's free access services—Internet Grateful Med and PubMed—you can search MEDLINE, the NLM's largest, most-used database, which offers more than 9 million selections from biomedical literature online. This is only one of more than 40 databases online, including more than 20 million records. Look through the latest literature on diseases, current research, consumer health information, special government programs, and publications. The NLM Web site is the sister site of the National Institutes of Health Web site.

Office of Minority Health Resource Center
P.O. Box 37337
Washington, DC 20013-7337
phone: 800-444-6472
TDD/TTY phone: 301-589-0951
fax: 301-589-0884
Web site: http://www.omhrc.gov

The Office of Minority Health Resource Center (OMHRC) is a nationwide service of the Office of Minority Health (OMH), which is part of the US Department of Health and Human Services Public Health Service. The OMH is dedicated to promoting the health of American Indian and Alaskan Native, African American, Asian and Pacific Islander, and Hispanic people. OMHRC answers requests for information on minority health concerns and provides referrals to appropriate organizations. Staff members can handle calls in both English and Spanish.

Social Security Administration
Office of Public Inquiries
6401 Security Blvd.
Baltimore, MD 21235-0001
phone: 800-772-1213 or 410-965-8882
TDD/TTY phone: 800-325-0778
Web site: http://www.ssa.gov

If you have a problem or need information or guidance, first contact your local Social Security Administration office or call one of the toll-free numbers listed above. Phone lines are open from 7:00 A.M. through 7:00 P.M. Monday through Friday (including the TDD/TTY phone line). The best times to call are mornings, evenings, at the end of the week, or toward the end of the month. If you have a touch-tone phone, recorded information and services are available 24 hours a day, including weekends and holidays. If you still need help, write to the Social Security Administration at the address above. Social Security Online is the official Web site of the Social Security Administration. The Web site offers useful information and guidance regarding Social Security benefits and services. You also can find your local Social Security office and access regional home pages through Social Security Online.

Veterans Affairs, Department of
Office of Consumer Affairs (075)
810 Vermont Ave., NW
Washington, DC 20420
phone: 800-827-1000
consumer affairs phone: 202-273-5771
Web site: http://www.va.gov

The Department of Veterans Affairs (VA) is the federal agency that oversees programs and provides benefits for military veterans and their dependents and beneficiaries. Benefits for eligible veterans include medical and dental care, vocational rehabilitation, and burial assistance. The publication *Federal Benefits for Veterans and Dependents* describes all the benefit programs and is available free from the VA.

Health Information Web Sites

Cancernet

Web site: http://cancernet.nci.nih.gov

CancerNet is an online information service provided by the National Cancer Institute, the federal agency that coordinates the government's cancer research programs. CancerNet provides access to up-to-date, accurate information about cancer that is continually reviewed and revised by cancer experts. Information available includes fact sheets, publications, and news about topics such as prevention, screening, detection, treatment, ongoing clinical trials, rehabilitation, and quality of life. CancerNet also provides access to PDQ, the National Cancer Institute's comprehensive cancer database and links to other National Cancer Institute home pages and organizations that offer cancer information, support services, and other helpful resources.

Caregiving Online

Web site: http://www.caregiving.com

Caregiving Online is an online support service from *Caregiving*, a monthly newsletter for caregivers (see page 186). This Web site provides an online support center, a caregivers' discussion group, a caregiving journal, a gallery of poems and essays by family caregivers, and links to other Web sites with valuable information and services for caregivers. Caregiving Online also provides access to hospice-related Web sites that offer support and helpful information on caring for people who are terminally ill.

ElderNet
Web site: http://www.eldernet.com

ElderNet is an online guide offering links to Web sites that deal with topics of interest to older people, including health, long-term care, legal assistance, financial planning, health and retirement benefits, specific diseases and conditions, alternative therapies, managed care, news, and entertainment. ElderNet's *Senior Lifestyles Directory* provides access to nationwide information about options such as retirement communities, assisted living, home care, and nursing facilities.

HealthFinder
Web site: http://www.healthfinder.gov

HealthFinder is a health information Web site for consumers developed by the US Department of Health and Human Services and other government agencies and coordinated by the Office of Disease Prevention and Health Promotion. Health-Finder gives you access to selected online publications, clearinghouses, databases, Web sites, support and self-help groups, government agencies, and nonprofit groups that produce reliable health-related information for consumers on a wide variety of health topics.

Information From Your Family Doctor
Web site: http://www.familydoctor.org

Information From Your Family Doctor is a patient-education Web site published by the American Academy of Family Physicians (AAFP). The AAFP is a national nonprofit medical association of family physicians, family practice residents, and medical students dedicated to promoting and maintaining quality standards for family doctors, who provide continuing comprehensive healthcare to the public. The information on the Web site is written and reviewed by physicians and patient education professionals at the AAFP and is reviewed and updated regularly. Consumers who access this site can locate useful information on hundreds of health topics of interest to women, men, children, and older people. You may search or browse the Web site for information on specific topics of interest to you.

Medem

Web site: http://www.medem.com

Medem, which stands for "medical empowerment," is made up of reliable content provided by the professional medical societies that are its members. This site is unique because it was founded by well-established professional organizations with proven experience. The content of the Web site is available to consumers either through Medem or via their own physician's secure Web site. Medem provides an experienced, credible, trusted source of healthcare information. It gives consumers the best healthcare information on the Internet and access to their doctors as well. The primary differences between Medem and other health Web sites are the quality and credentials of the healthcare information provided, and the delivery of this information via the Internet through individual physician Web sites. Medem provides various types of information, from peer-reviewed journal articles to medical news. Medem is an adjunct and tool to support the practice of medicine. It is not a replacement for direct patient-physician interaction. The societies that make up Medem do not see online interaction as a replacement for direct face-to-face interaction.

NetWellness

Web site: http://www.netwellness.org

NetWellness is an online health information service for consumers that was developed by the University of Cincinnati Medical Center, Case Western Reserve University, and Ohio State University. NetWellness offers up-to-date, general information on medications, diseases and conditions, standard and alternative treatments, and general health and wellness. The confidential and anonymous Ask an Expert feature allows you to get answers to your specific health questions. Most questions are answered within 1 to 2 days. NetWellness also provides links to other reliable, health-oriented Web sites.

Resource Directory for Older People

Web site: http://www.aoa.dhhs.gov/aoa/resource.html

The Resource Directory for Older People is an online guide to a wide array of organizations that offer valuable information and services of interest to older people, their families and caregivers, healthcare and legal professionals, social service providers, librarians, researchers, and the general public. The directory, which lists names, addresses, phone numbers, fax numbers, e-mail addresses, and Web sites, is provided through the cooperative efforts of the National Institute on Aging and the Administration on Aging, both of which are part of the US Department of Health and Human Services. The Resource Directory for Older People is continually updated. A printed version is available for $11.00 (prepaid with check or money order) by writing to: Superintendent of Documents; P.O. Box 371954; Pittsburgh, PA 15250-7954. Ask for publication number 0106200145-6. For credit card orders (VISA or MasterCard) call 202-512-1800.

RxList

Web site: http://www.rxlist.com

RxList is an online directory of more than 4,000 brand name and generic drugs. The directory includes drugs currently available in the United States or close to receiving approval from the US Food and Drug Administration. You can search for information on a specific drug or a category of drugs. Each entry provides a description of the generic drug and a list of brand names under which the drug is marketed. Other useful information includes indications (what the drug is used to treat), contraindications (when the drug should not be taken), warnings, precautions, drug interactions (other drugs or substances that can interfere with the drug's intended effects), adverse reactions (side effects), dosage, and estimated cost of therapy. RxList also includes a list of the 200 most-used drugs (for 1995, 1996, and 1997) based on data from prescriptions filled in the United States.

SeniorNet

121 Second St., 7th floor
San Francisco, CA 94105
phone: 415-495-4990
fax: 415-495-3999
Web site: http://www.seniornet.org

SeniorNet is a nonprofit educational organization that teaches older people (age 50 years and older) to use computers and the Internet. SeniorNet Learning Centers across the United States offer a wide variety of classes for both beginners and those who are more experienced with computers. Members are offered discounts on computer hardware, software, and other materials. Members also have access to SeniorNet Online, a nationwide computer network. SeniorNet publishes a newsletter, *Newsline*, and a variety of pamphlets on computer-related topics for older people.

Third Age

Web site: www.thirdage.com
Third Age is a Web site that provides access to a wide variety of

information, services, and other resources of interest to active older adults. Topics include healthy living, caregiving, retirement housing, family, and financial management. Third Age also offers chat rooms and forums in which older adults can express their views and share advice and experiences with others. Visitors to this Web site also will find online features such as a bookstore, news, and entertainment.

Home-Care Services and Hospice

Caregiving
Tad Publishing Company
P.O. Box 224
Park Ridge, IL 60068
phone: 847-823-0639
Web site: http://www.caregiving.com

Caregiving is a monthly newsletter that provides advice and support for people who are caring for an aging relative, friend, or neighbor. Caregivers will find valuable information on topics such as community services, emotional issues, skin care, lifting techniques, purchasing home medical equipment, hiring home health aides, and self-care. There is helpful advice tailored to the needs of employed caregivers, male caregivers, and caregivers of people who have dementia. Readers can submit questions to a team of home-care experts that includes two social workers, a home medical equipment supplier, a Medicare billing specialist, and dementia care specialists. Subscribers also have the opportunity to purchase products and services at a discount through the Caregivers Club.

Meals on Wheels Association of America
1414 Prince St., Suite 302
Alexandria, VA 22314

phone: 703-548-5558

fax: 703-548-8024

Web site: http://mowaa.org

Meals on Wheels programs deliver nutritious meals to people who are unable to leave home. You may call the national Meals on Wheels Association's toll-free number for additional information and to locate the Meals on Wheels program that serves your community.

National Alliance for Caregiving

4720 Montgomery Lane, Suite 642

Bethesda, MD 20814

phone: 301-718-8444

fax: 301-652-7711

Web site: http://www.caregiving.org

The National Alliance for Caregiving provides information and referral to national organizations that can help caregivers.

National Association for Home Care

228 Seventh St., SE

Washington, DC 20003

phone: 202-547-7424

fax: 202-547-3540

Web site: http://www.nahc.org

The National Association for Home Care (NAHC) is a trade organization that serves home-care agencies, hospices, and home-care aide organizations. The NAHC develops professional standards for home-care agencies, provides continuing education programs for home health aides, and monitors federal and state legislation pertaining to home care and hospice. The NAHC also provides listings of all local home-care agencies, information on the types of services they offer, and material on selecting a home-care agency. Consumers may access the Home

Care/Hospice Agency Locator on the NAHC Web site to locate home-care providers in their area.

National Caregiving Foundation
801 N. Pitt St., Room 116
Alexandria, VA 22314
phone: 703-299-9300
caregiver support kit request line: 800-930-1357
fax: 703-299-9304

The National Caregiving Foundation offers free information for caregivers of people who have Alzheimer's disease.

National Hospice and Palliative Care Organization
1700 Diagonal Rd., Suite 300
Alexandria, VA 22314
phone: 800-658-8898 or 703-243-5900
Web site: http://www.nhpco.org

The National Hospice and Palliative Care Organization (NHPCO) is a private, nonprofit group dedicated to promoting and maintaining compassionate, quality care for people who are terminally ill and their families. The NHPCO also works to educate the general public and healthcare professionals about hospice and to make hospice care an integral part of the US healthcare system. The NHPCO publishes *The Guide to the Nation's Hospices*, a comprehensive listing of hospices across the United States. Consumers may call the NHPCO toll-free number for referrals to local hospice programs. The NHPCO also maintains a comprehensive library of materials (including books, directories, audiotapes, and videotapes) related to hospice for its members. Various publications and hospice-related products are available for sale through the NHPCO store.

Visiting Nurse Associations of America
11 Beacon St., Suite 910

Boston, MA 02108
phone: 617-523-4042
fax: 617-227-4843
Web site: http://www.vnaa.org/home.htm

The Visiting Nurse Associations of America (VNAA) is the official, national association of freestanding, not-for-profit, community-based visiting nurse agencies. The VNAA is committed to providing effective, innovative, and personalized community-based home healthcare. Through its Web site, VNAA offers advice on choosing a visiting nurse agency and provides answers to commonly asked questions about home care. The VNAA Referral System can help you locate a visiting nurse agency in your area.

Long-Term Care and Housing

American Association of Homes and Services for the Aging
901 E St., NW, Suite 500
Washington, DC 20004-2011
phone: 202-783-2242
fax: 202-783-2255
Web site: http://www.aahsa.org

The American Association of Homes and Services for the Aging (AAHSA) is a trade association that represents more than 5,000 nonprofit nursing facilities, continuing-care retirement communities, senior housing facilities, and community service providers. The AAHSA provides consumer-oriented information on long-term care and housing options such as continuing-care retirement communities, nursing homes, and assisted living facilities. This information can help you to determine your needs and then locate and evaluate accredited facilities and services.

Assisted Living Federation of America
10300 Eaton Pl., Suite 400
Fairfax, VA 22030
phone: 703-691-8100
fax: 703-691-8106
Web site: http://www.alfa.org

The Assisted Living Federation of America (ALFA) is a trade association devoted to promoting the interests of assisted living providers (assisted living facilities and related organizations) and enhancing the quality of life of people who reside in assisted living facilities. The ALFA offers consumers a list of assisted living residences by state and a free consumer brochure and checklist that contains information on how to choose and evaluate these facilities.

National Citizens' Coalition for Nursing Home Reform
1424 16th St., NW, Suite 202
Washington, DC 20036-2211
phone: 202-332-2275
fax: 202-332-2949
Web site: http://www.nccnhr.org

The National Citizens' Coalition for Nursing Home Reform is a nationwide consumer-advocacy group that works to ensure the quality of long-term care services. The coalition achieves its goals through consumer information and education; advocacy; citizen action groups; ombudsman programs; and enforcement of consumer-directed health, living, and care-delivery standards. The National Citizens' Coalition for Nursing Home Reform is home to the National Long-Term Care Ombudsman Resources Center, which also serves as a clearinghouse for current information on institution-based long-term care. Consumers may request a list of publications available for sale.

Support Housing for the Elderly

Programs offered through the US Department of Housing and Urban Development (HUD) can help older people find affordable housing. For information, contact your local HUD office, listed in the blue pages of your local telephone directory.

Mental Health

American Academy of Child and Adolescent Psychiatry
3615 Wisconsin Ave., NW
Washington, DC 20016-3007
phone: 202-966-7300
fax: 202-966-2891
Web site: http://www.aacap.org

The American Academy of Child and Adolescent Psychiatry (AACAP) is a nonprofit organization with more than 6,500 members (mostly psychiatrists and other physicians). The academy is the leading national professional medical association dedicated to treating and improving the quality of life for children and adolescents affected by mental, behavioral, and developmental disorders, and their families. The Web site provides information on child and adolescent psychiatry, press releases, information on legislation and meetings, fact sheets for parents and caregivers, membership, research, and clinical practice guidelines. Its mission is to promote mentally healthy children and adolescents through research, training, advocacy, prevention, diagnosis and treatment, and peer support and collaboration.

American Association of Suicidology
4201 Connecticut Ave., NW, Suite 408
Washington, DC 20008
phone: 202-237-2280

fax: 202-237-2282

Web site: http://www.suicidology.org

The American Association of Suicidology (AAS) is a nonprofit organization dedicated to the understanding and prevention of suicide. The AAS promotes research, public awareness programs, education, and training for mental health professionals, suicide survivors, students, and volunteers. The association develops certification standards for suicide prevention and crisis centers and evaluates crisis workers for certification in crisis management. The AAS serves as a national clearinghouse for information on suicide. Publications include *Suicide and Life-Threatening Behavior*, a quarterly journal; *Newslink*, a quarterly newsletter for members; and *Surviving Suicide*, a quarterly newsletter for survivors. The AAS membership is open to mental health organizations, mental health professionals, students, volunteers, and anyone with an interest in suicide prevention or life-threatening behaviors. Contact AAS for free information on suicide and suicide prevention and nationwide referrals to suicide prevention and crisis centers and support groups.

American Psychiatric Association

1400 K St., NW

Washington, DC 20005

phone: 888-357-7924

fax: 202-682-6850

Web site: http://www.psych.org

The American Psychiatric Association (APA) is a professional organization of physicians who specialize in psychiatry. The association offers information on mental health issues and referrals to state psychiatric societies, which can make referrals to local psychiatrists. The APA Web site offers online versions of two types of APA pamphlets for consumers: *Let's Talk Facts About* and *APA Fact Sheets*. Topics available online include

Alzheimer's disease, depression, coping with HIV and AIDS, substance abuse, teen suicide, counseling after disasters, and memories of sexual abuse. For a complete list of available pamphlets and for information on ordering hard-copy versions, access the APA Web site, or send your request to the association at the address above.

American Psychological Association
750 First St., NE
Washington, DC 20002-4242
phone: 800-374-2721 or 202-336-5500
Web site: http://www.apa.org

The American Psychological Association (APA) is the world's largest association of psychologists. The APA works for the advancement of psychology as a science, as a profession, and as a means of promoting human welfare. It provides free referrals to local practitioners nationwide. In addition, the APA publishes a variety of brochures and pamphlets on mental health topics of interest to consumers, including *Breast Cancer: How Your Mind Can Help Your Body*, *Controlling Anger—Before It Controls You*, and *Managing Traumatic Stress: Tips for Recovering From Disasters and Other Traumatic Events*. The association also publishes a series of children's books on a wide variety of topics to help children deal with the problems they confront while growing up. Topics include adoption and foster care, depression, divorce, school problems, and self-esteem. Contact APA for a referral or for more information about obtaining publications.

AMI Québec
5253 Decarie Blvd., Suite 150
Montréal, Québec, Canada H3W 3C3
phone: 514-486-1448
fax: 514-486-6157
Web site: http://www.dsuper.net/~amique

AMI Québec (Alliance for the Mentally Ill, Inc.) is a grassroots support and advocacy group that serves the families and friends of people who are mentally ill. AMI Québec works to eliminate the stigma occasionally associated with mental illness by raising public awareness. AMI Québec offers a variety of self-help groups, seminars, education programs, and other resources, mainly for the English-speaking population. AMI Québec also advocates legislation for protection of and quality care for people with mental illness and promotes research on treatment, rehabilitation, and cure.

National Alliance for the Mentally Ill
Colonial Place Three
2107 Wilson Blvd., Suite 300
Arlington, VA 22201-3042
phone: 703-524-7600
helpline phone: 800-950-NAMI (800-950-6264)
TDD/TTY phone: 703-516-7227
fax: 703-524-9094
Web site: http://www.nami.org

Founded in 1979, the National Alliance for the Mentally Ill (NAMI) is a nonprofit self-help support group made up of family and friends of people with mental illness. It is an advocacy organization dedicated solely to improving the lives of people with schizophrenia, bipolar disorder, severe depression, obsessive-compulsive disorder, and severe anxiety disorders. The 210,000 members of NAMI seek equitable services for people with severe psychiatric illness. It provides information about severe brain disorders and supports increased funding for research and adequate health insurance, housing, rehabilitation, and jobs. The NAMI helpline provides referrals to support groups in your area and answers to questions about mental health.

National Institute of Mental Health
Public Inquiries
6001 Executive Blvd., Room 8184, MSC-9663
Bethesda, MD 20892-9663
phone: 301-443-4513
fax: 301-443-4279
Web site: http://www.nimh.nih.gov

The National Institute of Mental Health (NIMH) is part of the National Institutes of Health (NIH), the principal biomedical and behavioral research agency of the US government. The NIH is part of the US Department of Health and Human Services. The NIMH is dedicated to achieving better understanding, treatment, and prevention of mental illness through research. A wide variety of brochures, information sheets, reports, press releases, fact sheets, and other educational materials that contain the latest information about symptoms, diagnosis, and treatment of various mental illnesses are available from the NIMH. Topics include anxiety disorders, bipolar disorder, depression, learning disabilities, obsessive-compulsive disorder, and many others. Access this and other useful information on the NIMH Web site or call or write NIMH for additional information.

Rehabilitation

American Physical Therapy Association
Section on Geriatrics
1111 N. Fairfax St.
Alexandria, VA 22314-1488
phone: 703-684-APTA (703-684-2782)
fax: 703-684-7343
Web site: http://www.geriatricspt.org/consumer/ggeneral.html

The American Physical Therapy Association (APTA) is a professional organization dedicated to the advancement of physical therapy practice, research, and education. The APTA Section on Geriatrics offers helpful information for older consumers, including an overview of physical therapy and its potential benefits, a state-by-state listing of physical therapists who have been certified as geriatric specialists by APTA, and other resources (such as exercise tips, guidelines for taking care of your back, and advice on dealing with incontinence).

National Rehabilitation Information Center
1010 Wayne Ave., Suite 800
Silver Springs, MD 20910
phone: 800-346-2742 or 301-562-2400
TDD/TTY phone: 301-495-5626
fax: 301-562-2401
Web site: http://www.naric.com/naric

The National Rehabilitation Information Center (NARIC) is funded by the National Institute on Disability and Rehabilitation Research of the US Department of Education. The NARIC provides information and referral services for anyone interested in mental and physical disability and rehabilitation and strives to make all of its products and services accessible to all US citizens. You may call, write, or visit the facility in person to request information and referrals at no cost. The NARIC has an extensive collection of publications that includes books, journal articles, pamphlets, audiovisuals, and more. The NARIC can perform database searches for materials on specific topics and provide photocopies of those materials (within the limits of current US copyright law). Most NARIC publications (including materials obtained through database searches) are also available in large-print, audiocassette, and braille format; all NARIC documents are available on PC-compatible disks.

Self-help and Support

American Self-help Clearinghouse
100 Hanover Ave., 2nd Floor
Cedar Knolls, NJ 07927
phone: 973-326-6789
fax: 973-326-9467
Web site: http://www.selfhelpgroups.org

The American Self-help Clearinghouse offers access to information on more than 800 national and international self-help and support groups through its searchable online database, Self-help Sourcebook Online. The clearinghouse also publishes a hard-copy version, *Self-help Sourcebook*, which is available for purchase by mail. Visit the Web site to access Self-help Sourcebook Online.

Catholic Golden Age
National Headquarters
RD#2, Box 161
Olyphant, PA 18447
phone: 800-836-5699 or 570-586-1091
fax: 570-586-7721
Web site: http://www.catholicgoldenage.org

Catholic Golden Age is a charitable organization that helps older people meet their physical, intellectual, social, economic, and spiritual needs. The organization offers group insurance plans and discounts on eyeglasses, prescriptions, and travel to its members. Programs conducted by local chapters include health promotion and disease prevention. Catholic Golden Age also publishes *CGA World*, a bimonthly newsletter.

Children of Aging Parents
1609 Woodbourne Rd., Suite 302-A

Levittown, PA 19057
phone: 800-227-7294 or 215-945-6900
fax: 215-945-8720
Web site: http://www.careguide.net/careguide.cgi/caps/
  capshome.html

Children of Aging Parents (CAPS) is a nonprofit membership organization for people who are caring for aging relatives. CAPS conducts workshops for community groups to promote understanding of the special needs of older people and offers training programs for nurses and social workers in hospitals, nursing facilities, and rehabilitation centers. CAPS is a clearinghouse for information on resources for older people; call its information and referral service to learn about support groups and other resources available in your community. CAPS publishes a newsletter, *Capsule*, for members, and produces brochures and fact sheets for caregivers.

Choice in Dying
National Office
1035 30th St., NW
Washington, DC 20007
phone: 800-989-WILL (800-989-9455)
  or 202-338-9790
fax: 202-338-0242
Web site: http://www.choices.org

Choice in Dying is a nonprofit organization that assists patients and their families with end-of-life medical care decision-making. The organization provides state-specific living will and health-care proxy (durable power of attorney for healthcare) forms for a nominal fee, counsels patients and their families, educates and advises through its publications and training and outreach programs, and supports patients' rights legislation at state and federal levels.

Disabled American Veterans
National Service and Legislative Headquarters
807 Maine Ave., SW
Washington, DC 20024
phone: 202-554-3501
Web site: http://www.dav.org

Disabled American Veterans (DAV) is a private, nonprofit organization dedicated to serving veterans who have service-related disabilities and their families. Services provided include counseling, employment programs, help in obtaining free healthcare, and assistance with filing claims for veterans' benefits such as disability compensation and pensions. The Older Veterans Assistance Program offers additional assistance to older veterans and their families. A list of free publications is available from your state DAV service office; check your local phone book or call the number listed above to locate the DAV office that serves your state.

Friends Health Connection
P.O. Box 114
New Brunswick, NJ 08903
phone: 800-483-7436
fax: 732-249-9897
Web site: http://www.48friend.org

For a modest fee, Friends Health Connection (a nonprofit organization) matches people who have health problems—whether a disease, condition, disability, or injury—with other people who have similar health problems, for friendship and support. Friends Health Connection's Family Network provides a similar service for caregivers, family members, and friends of people who have health problems. You or your loved one can establish such a relationship via mail, telephone, or e-mail.

National Easter Seal Society
230 W. Monroe St., Suite 1800
Chicago, IL 60606
phone: 800-221-6827 or 312-726-6200
TDD/TTY phone: 312-726-4258
fax: 312-726-1494
Web site: http://www.easter-seals.org

The National Easter Seal Society (Easter Seals) is a nationwide, community-based organization that serves children and adults with disabilities and their families. Easter Seals provides services such as preschool, day care, after-school care, camp, respite care, job training, job placement, mentoring, medical screening, rehabilitation, and support.

National Self-help Clearinghouse
Web site: http://www.selfhelpweb.org

The National Self-help Clearinghouse provides information about and referrals to self-help groups nationwide. The clearinghouse offers technical assistance, advice, and training programs to established self-help groups and also offers guidance to people who want to organize self-help groups. A list of clearinghouse publications also is available.

Self Help for Hard of Hearing People, Inc.
7910 Woodmont Ave., Suite 1200
Bethesda, MD 20814
phone: 301-657-2248
TDD/TTY phone: 301-657-2249
fax: 301-913-9413
Web site: http://www.shhh.org

Self Help for Hard of Hearing People, Inc. (SHHH) is an organization that works to improve quality of life for people with impaired hearing through education, advocacy, and self-help. SHHH publishes a quarterly newsletter, *SHHH News*, and a bimonthly magazine, *Hearing Loss: The Journal of Self Help for Hard of Hearing People*. SHHH provides guidance and support for older people, adults, young adults, teens, children, and parents of children with hearing loss. In addition, SHHH offers consumers and professionals a wide variety of publications on topics related to hearing loss, including prevention, detection, coping, hearing aids, and effective communication, and the *SHHH Information Series*, books, pamphlets, reports, videotapes, audiotapes, and posters. Local chapters of SHHH offer support and encouragement to people with hearing loss and provide information about and referrals to community resources.

Well Spouse Foundation
30 E. 40th St., PH
New York, NY 10016
phone: 800-838-0879 or 212-685-8815
fax: 212-685-8676
Web site: http://www.wellspouse.org

Well Spouse Foundation is a nonprofit self-help organization that offers support for people who are caring for a chronically ill or disabled spouse. The organization helps to educate health-care professionals, politicians, and the general public about long-term care and the needs of caregivers. Well Spouse Foundation publishes a bimonthly newsletter, *Mainstay*, and sponsors an annual weekend conference for its members. The organization also provides personal outreach to its members through calls and letters and ongoing support for members whose spouses have died.

Miscellaneous

Alliance of Claims Assistance Professionals
731 Naperville Rd.

Wheaton, IL 60187-6407
phone: 630-588-1260
fax: 630-690-0377
e-mail: askus@claims.org
Web site: http://www.claims.org

The Alliance of Claims Assistance Professionals is a national, nonprofit professional organization that can help you locate experienced professionals in your area who can assist you with processing health insurance claims.

CenterWatch, Inc.

22 Thomson Place, 36T1
Boston, MA 02210-1212
editorial office phone: 617-856-5900
editorial office fax: 617-856-5901 or 800-850-1232
subscriber services phone: 800-765-9647
subscriber services fax: 800-850-1232
Web site: http://www.centerwatch.com

CenterWatch, Inc., is a clinical trials listing service from which you can get information about clinical trials and newly approved drugs, including generic equivalents, that are on the market. You can search the Web site for a particular clinical trial, be notified via e-mail about new trials recruiting participants, and read about medical centers that are conducting research.

Job Accommodation Network

West Virginia University
P.O. Box 6080
Morgantown, WV 26506-6080
phone: 800-526-7234
Web site: http://janweb.icdi.wvu.edu

The Job Accommodation Network is an international toll-free consulting service that provides information about job accommodations for employing people with disabilities as well as general employer and employee information.

Medic Alert Foundation
2323 Colorado Ave.
Turlock, CA 95382-2018
phone: 800-IDALERT (800-432-5378)
fax: 209-669-2450
Web site: http://www.medicalert.org

Medic Alert is a nonprofit membership organization that provides identification and medical information in emergencies. Each member wears an identification bracelet or pendant bearing an emblem that indicates the wearer has a hidden medical condition and/or needs special medical treatment in emergency situations. He or she also carries a wallet card that contains up-to-date personal medical information. The emblem alerts emergency workers and others to vital medical facts about the person and instructs them to contact a 24-hour emergency response center where trained personnel provide lifesaving information. Medic Alert bracelets and pendants are particularly helpful for people with allergies, chronic conditions (such as diabetes or epilepsy), or implants; people who take medications; or people with Parkinson's disease or Alzheimer's disease. Medic Alert charges a modest yearly fee for membership.

National Center for Complementary and Alternative Medicine Clearinghouse
P.O. Box 8218
Silver Springs, MD 20907-8218
phone: 888-644-6226
TTY/TDY phone: 888-644-6226
fax: 301-495-4957
e-mail: nccamc@altmedinfo.org

Web site: http://nccam.nih.gov

The National Center for Complementary and Alternative Medicine (NCCAM) disseminates information to the public, media, and healthcare professionals to promote awareness and education about complementary and alternative medicine research. The stated purpose of NCCAM is to facilitate the evaluation of alternative medical treatment to determine its effectiveness. NCCAM meets with the US Food and Drug Administration to reevaluate current rules and regulations concerning research on, and the use of, devices, equipment, herbs, and homeopathic remedies. The center conducts research; it does not serve as a referral agency for alternative medical treatments or for individual practitioners. Inclusion of a treatment in its literature or Web site does not imply endorsement by NCCAM. NCCAM cautions people not to seek the therapies without the consultation of a licensed healthcare provider.

Office on Smoking and Health

National Center for Chronic Disease Prevention and Health
Promotion Centers for Disease Control and Prevention
Mail Stop K-50
4770 Buford Hwy., NE
Atlanta, GA 30341-3717
phone: 800-CDC-1311 (800-232-1311) or 770-488-5705
automated fax information service: 888-232-3299
Web site: http://www.cdc.gov/tobacco

The National Center for Chronic Disease Prevention and Health Promotion offers a wide variety of materials and information that are useful for people with high blood pressure. The Office on Smoking and Health provides publications on smoking and health and information on quitting smoking.

Glossary

This glossary defines terms that your doctor may have used or that you may have read or heard. Italicized terms within definitions refer you to other terms in the glossary for additional information.

A

ACE inhibitor   Angiotensin-converting enzyme inhibitor. An *antihypertensive* used to treat *high blood pressure* and *heart failure*.

acid reflux   The backflow of acid from the stomach into the esophagus (the muscular tube that connects the throat with the stomach) caused by a defective valve at the entrance to the stomach.

ADHD   See *attention-deficit hyperactivity disorder.*

adrenal glands   A pair of triangular glands located directly above each *kidney*. Produce a variety of *hormones* that affect nearly every system in the body.

adrenaline   See *epinephrine.*

advance directive   A legal document designed to help ensure that healthcare decisions made on a person's behalf are consistent with his or her preferences. See also *do-not-resuscitate order, durable power of attorney for healthcare,* and *living will.*

aerobic exercise   A physical exercise that requires the heart and lungs to work harder to meet the muscles' continuous demand for oxygen. Examples include brisk walking, dancing, step aerobics, jogging, and biking.

AFP test   Alpha-fetoprotein test. A blood test performed on pregnant women between the 15th and 18th weeks of pregnancy to measure the level of alpha-fetoprotein (AFP), a *protein* produced by the fetus and found in amniotic fluid (the clear fluid that surrounds a fetus during pregnancy). An elevated blood level of AFP may indicate abnormalities such as *neural tube defects* in the fetus. AFP is also used in a test to detect a type of liver tumor and cancer of the testicle.

AIDS Acquired immunodeficiency syndrome. A disorder of the *immune system* caused by infection with *HIV*.

allergen Any substance—such as pollen, animal dander, or a particular food—that produces an *allergic reaction* in some people.

allergic contact dermatitis A skin condition that occurs when the skin comes in contact with an *allergen*, causing a rash that is characterized by redness, swelling, and blisters. May be difficult to distinguish from other skin conditions. See also *eczema, atopic*.

allergic reaction An inappropriate *immune system* response that occurs when an *allergen* enters the body.

allergy An abnormal sensitivity to an *allergen*.

alpha blocker A medication used to treat heart and circulation disorders such as *high blood pressure* and *peripheral vascular disease*.

ALS Amyotrophic lateral sclerosis; also called Lou Gehrig's disease. The most common *motor neuron disease*, characterized by a progressive loss of muscle function that leads to paralysis.

Alzheimer's disease A progressive, incurable condition that destroys brain cells and gradually causes loss of intellectual abilities such as memory and extreme changes in personality and behavior.

amino acids Chemical compounds that are the basic components of all *proteins*.

amnesia Loss of the ability to store information in memory or to recall information already stored in memory. Can be caused by brain damage or disease and is a common symptom of various neurological disorders.

amniocentesis A diagnostic procedure performed on pregnant women in which a small amount of amniotic fluid (the clear fluid that surrounds a fetus during pregnancy) is removed with a needle and examined in a laboratory. Performed to detect abnormalities in a fetus.

anabolic steroids Synthetic drugs that imitate the effects of *testosterone*.

anaphylactic shock A severe, life-threatening *allergic reaction* that requires immediate medical treatment. Symptoms include a sudden, severe drop in *blood pressure* and difficulty breathing.

anemia A blood disorder caused by a deficiency of red blood cells or *hemoglobin*. Reduces the ability of the blood to supply oxygen to the tissues and to remove carbon dioxide from the body.

aneurysm An abnormal ballooning of a weakened area in an *artery* wall. An aneurysm in the brain may rupture, causing a hemorrhagic *stroke*.

angina A tight, heavy, squeezing sensation of pain deep beneath the breastbone or in a band across the chest that results from a reduced supply of oxygen to the heart muscle, indicating *heart disease*. The pain also may radiate to the left arm, shoulder, neck, jaw, or middle of the back and may be accompanied by nausea, sweating, or shortness of breath.

angiography A diagnostic procedure for examining the inside of an *artery*. A *contrast medium* is injected through a *catheter* into the artery, and a rapid-sequence series of X rays is taken.

angioplasty A surgical procedure used to clear a narrowed or blocked *artery*.

anorexia A potentially life-threatening eating disorder (most frequent in young women) that is characterized by an abnormal fear of being fat, prolonged avoidance of food, excessive weight loss, and obsession with exercise.

antibiotic A medication used to treat bacterial infections.

antibodies Also called immunoglobulins. *Proteins* found in the blood and tissue fluids that protect the body from infectious organisms.

anticoagulant A medication used to treat abnormal blood clotting.

antidepressant A medication used to treat *depression*. Three commonly prescribed types of antidepressants are tricyclic antidepressants, monoamine oxidase inhibitors, and selective *serotonin* reuptake inhibitors.

antihistamine A medication that blocks the effects of *histamine*.

antihypertensive A medication used to treat *high blood pressure*. See also *ACE inhibitor, beta blocker, calcium channel blocker,* and *diuretic*.

anti-inflammatory A medication such as aspirin or ibuprofen that relieves the symptoms of inflammation.

antioxidant A compound that protects against cell damage caused by *free radicals*.

aorta The body's main *artery*.

aortic stenosis The most common heart valve disorder. Causes narrowing or stiffening of the *aortic valve* and can lead to *angina* and *heart failure*.

aortic valve The valve between the *aorta* and the left *ventricle* of the heart.

arrhythmia An abnormally fast or slow *heartbeat* or an irregular heartbeat.

arteriole A tiny branch of an *artery*.

arteriosclerosis A term used to describe a group of disorders characterized by thickening and scarring of *artery* walls. See also *atherosclerosis*.

artery A blood vessel that carries oxygen-filled blood away from the heart to the organs and tissues.

arthritis A general term used to describe inflammation of a *joint* accompanied by swelling, stiffness, and pain. See also *osteoarthritis* and *rheumatoid arthritis*.

arthroplasty A surgical procedure in which a damaged joint is replaced with an artificial joint made of metal and plastic. Most often performed on the knee and hip but also performed on the ankles, hands, wrists, and toes.

arthroscopy   Examination of or surgery on a *joint* using a viewing tube called an arthroscope inserted through a small incision.

asthma   A respiratory disorder characterized by reversible narrowing of the airways, causing wheezing, shortness of breath, chest tightness, and coughing.

asymptomatic   Without signs or symptoms of disease.

atheroma   Fatty deposits on the inner lining of an *artery* that can lead to *atherosclerosis*.

atherosclerosis   The buildup of fatty material called arterial plaque (see *plaque, arterial*) in the inner lining of an *artery*. Can narrow the blood vessels and reduce blood flow to the organs and tissues, increasing the risk of a *heart attack* or *stroke*.

athlete's foot   Also called tinea pedis. A common contagious fungal infection of the foot that affects the skin between the toes or on the soles or sides of the feet. Causes the skin to itch, peel, crack, and, occasionally, form blisters.

atrial fibrillation   An abnormal *heartbeat* in which the *atria* beat rapidly and irregularly and independently of the *ventricles*.

atrium   One of the two small upper chambers of the heart.

attention-deficit hyperactivity disorder   A behavior problem in which a person is hyperactive, easily distracted, has difficulty paying attention and completing tasks, and acts impulsively. People who have this disorder may also have learning disabilities.

audiogram   A graphic record of a person's hearing ability that is obtained during *audiometry*.

audiometry   Hearing tests performed to measure a person's ability to hear.

autism   A developmental disorder that affects the functioning of the brain, resulting in impaired emotional, social, and language development. Of unknown cause.

autoimmune disease   A disease in which the *immune system* mistakenly attacks the body's own cells and tissues.

autologous blood donation   Donation of a person's own blood before scheduled elective surgery to make the blood available in case a transfusion is necessary during or after surgery.

B

basal cell carcinoma   A slow-growing form of skin cancer, found in the outer layer of skin, that rarely spreads to other parts of the body. Accounts for about 90 percent of all skin cancers.

Bell's palsy   A peripheral nerve disorder that causes one-sided weakness, twitching, or paralysis of the facial muscles.

benign   Not cancerous.

benign prostatic hyperplasia Noncancerous enlargement of the *prostate gland* that obstructs the flow and passage of urine through the *urethra*.

beta blocker An *antihypertensive* used to treat heart and circulation disorders such as *angina, high blood pressure,* and *arrhythmia.*

beta carotene An *antioxidant* found in orange and deep yellow fruits and vegetables that converts into vitamin A in the body.

bile A greenish liquid that the liver secretes to remove waste products and aid in the digestion of fat.

biopsy A diagnostic test in which a small sample of tissue is removed from the body and examined under a microscope.

bipolar disorder Also called manic-depressive disorder. A mood disorder characterized by alternating episodes of deep *depression* and euphoria.

blood clot A clump of coagulated blood.

blood pressure A measure of the force exerted against the walls of the *arteries* by the flow of blood as it is pumped through the body by the heart. Systolic pressure is the first, higher number in a blood pressure reading, indicating the pressure in the blood vessels when the heart beats and pumps blood through the arteries. Diastolic pressure is the second, lower number that indicates the pressure in the blood vessels when the heart rests between beats and fills with blood.

BMI See *body mass index.*

body mass index A measurement used to determine whether a person's body weight is in the healthful range.

bone density A measure of the amount of *calcium* and other minerals in bone in relation to the width of the bone. Used to determine a person's risk of developing *osteoporosis.*

botulism An often fatal form of *food poisoning* that usually results from eating improperly preserved or canned foods.

brachytherapy A type of *radiation therapy* in which the source of radiation is placed near the surface of the body or inserted into a body cavity or tissue. Brachytherapy is sometimes used to treat cancer of the *prostate gland.*

bradycardia A *heart rate* below 60 beats per minute.

bulimia An eating disorder characterized by binge overeating followed by self-induced vomiting or laxative abuse.

bursa A fluid-filled sac that acts as a cushion at a pressure point in the body, often near a *joint.*

bursitis Inflammation of a *bursa* that can result from *arthritis,* injury, or infection.

C

CA-125 test Cancer antigen test. A test used to determine the blood level of CA-125, a protein made by cancer cells, to help diagnose ovarian cancer in women. An elevated level of CA-125 may indicate ovarian cancer but can also be a sign of *fibroids* or of a gastrointestinal disorder.

calcitonin   A *hormone* produced by the *thyroid gland* that helps control the level of calcium in the blood and enhance bone formation. Sometimes used to help prevent *osteoporosis*.

calcium   A mineral that is important for strong bones and teeth and also has an important role in muscle contraction, blood clotting, and nerve function.

calcium channel blocker   An *antihypertensive* used to treat heart and circulation disorders such as *angina* and *high blood pressure*.

campylobacter poisoning   A form of *food poisoning* from consuming undercooked poultry, raw milk, or water that is contaminated with the campylobacter bacterium.

candidiasis   A common yeast infection that occurs most often in the vagina and, in children, in the mouth. Candidiasis also can occur in people whose *immune systems* are weakened by a virus such as *HIV* or a disease such as *AIDS*.

capillaries   Tiny blood vessels.

carcinogen   Any substance, such as cigarette smoke, that can cause cancer.

cardiac catheterization   A diagnostic procedure in which a *catheter* is threaded through a blood vessel into the heart to monitor its function and to inject *contrast medium* for imaging.

cardiopulmonary resuscitation   See *CPR*.

cardiovascular system   Also called the circulatory system. The network formed by the heart and blood vessels that pumps blood and carries it throughout the body.

carotid artery   One of the four major *arteries* that supply blood to the head and neck.

carotid endarterectomy   A surgical procedure to remove arterial plaque (see *plaque, arterial*) from the *carotid arteries*.

carpal tunnel syndrome   A common *repetitive stress injury* characterized by numbness, tingling, and pain in the wrist and hand. Caused by compression of a nerve where it enters the hand.

cartilage   A type of *connective tissue* that is an important structural component of certain parts of the skeletal system such as the *joints*.

cataract   A cloudy area in the normally clear lens of the eye that causes impaired vision.

catheter   A thin, flexible tube that is inserted into a vessel or body cavity to withdraw or instill fluids or to widen a passageway.

cauterize   To burn with a hot instrument or caustic chemical to destroy tissue, stop bleeding, or promote healing.

chemotherapy   Treatment of cancer using powerful drugs to destroy cancer cells throughout the body.

chlamydia   The most common *sexually transmitted disease;* caused by the microorganism Chlamydia trachomatis. Women usually do not have symptoms, while men usually have burning during urination, a clear discharge from the penis, and swelling or pain in the testicles.

cholesterol   A fatlike substance that is an important component of cells and is involved in the transport of fats in the blood. High-density lipoprotein (HDL) cholesterol (the "good" cholesterol) protects against *heart disease* by cleansing blood vessels of low-density lipoprotein (LDL) cholesterol (the "bad" cholesterol). LDL cholesterol increases the risk of *atherosclerosis* and heart disease.

chromosomal disorders   Diseases or conditions caused by abnormalities in the number or structure of *chromosomes.* Some are inherited but most occur by chance during conception.

chromosome   Threadlike structures inside the nucleus of a cell that contain *genes.* Body cells have 46 chromosomes; egg and sperm cells have 23.

circulatory system   See *cardiovascular system.*

coccidian infection   A form of *food poisoning* caused by microorganisms that can be found in unpasteurized apple cider, raw fruits and vegetables, and contaminated water.

colitis   Inflammation of the *colon.*

colon   The main section of the large intestine.

colonoscopy   An examination of the *colon* using a long, flexible viewing instrument called a colonoscope.

colostomy   A surgical procedure in which part of the *colon* is brought through an incision in the abdominal wall and an artificial opening is created through which feces can be discharged into a bag attached to the skin.

computed tomography scan   See *CT scan.*

conductive hearing loss   Impaired hearing caused by inadequate transmission of sound from the outer ear to the inner ear.

congenital   Present from birth.

congestive heart failure   See *heart failure.*

connective tissue   A type of tissue, such as *cartilage* and *tendons,* that holds various body structures together.

contrast medium   A type of dye that is injected into an artery during diagnostic procedures such as *angiography* and *ERCP.*

cornea   The tough, transparent, dome-shaped covering at the front of the eyeball that protects the eye and helps focus light onto the *retina.*

coronary artery bypass   A surgical procedure in which additional blood vessels are grafted onto obstructed coronary *arteries* to allow blood to flow around (bypass) the obstructed areas and reach the heart.

coronary artery disease See *heart disease.*

corticosteroids Medications that imitate the actions of the natural *hormones* secreted by the *adrenal glands.* These drugs have many uses, including treatment of inflammatory disorders such as *arthritis, asthma, allergic contact dermatitis,* and *tendinitis.*

CPR Cardiopulmonary resuscitation. A lifesaving procedure in which cardiac massage and artificial ventilation are performed on a person whose heart has stopped beating. Performed to maintain the circulation of oxygenated blood to the brain.

Crohn's disease A chronic, inflammatory disease of the digestive tract. Of unknown cause.

cryotherapy Also called cryosurgery. A procedure that uses low temperatures (such as those of liquid nitrogen) to destroy abnormal tissue by freezing.

CT scan Computed tomography scan. A diagnostic technique that uses a computer and low-dose X rays to produce detailed cross-sectional images of body tissues that are displayed on a video monitor.

cyanosis Bluish coloring of the skin and *mucous membranes* caused by inadequate oxygen in the blood.

cyst An abnormal lump or swelling that is filled with fluid.

cystitis Inflammation of the inner lining of the bladder, usually caused by bacterial infection.

cystoscopy Examination of the bladder and ureters (tubes that carry urine from the *kidneys* to the bladder) using a viewing tube called a cystoscope.

cytomegalovirus A type of *herpesvirus* that can cause serious illness in people with weakened *immune systems* such as people with *AIDS.*

D

D and C Dilation and curettage. A surgical procedure that involves dilation (widening) of the cervix and curettage (scraping) of the endometrium (the membrane that lines the uterus). Used to diagnose and treat disorders of the uterus such as heavy, persistent vaginal bleeding.

deep-vein thrombosis Formation of *blood clots* in *veins* deep inside the legs. Usually results from sluggish blood flow caused by lack of activity.

defibrillator A device that restores a normal *heartbeat* by delivering a brief electric shock to the heart muscle.

delirium Sudden, temporary mental confusion.

dementia Progressive, permanent decline in mental abilities.

depression A mood disorder characterized by feelings of sadness, hopelessness, and helplessness combined with apathy, poor self-esteem, and withdrawal from social situations.

dermatitis   See *allergic contact dermatitis*.

desensitization   A technique used to treat *phobias* in which a person is gradually exposed to the object or situation that he or she fears.

diabetes   A disorder in which the body is unable to make or use *insulin* properly. There are two major forms: type 1 and type 2. Type 1 is an *autoimmune disease* in which the immune system attacks the cells of the *pancreas* that produce insulin. In type 2, which is the most common form of diabetes, the body's cells gradually fail to respond to insulin.

diabetic retinopathy   Damage to the blood vessels of the *retina*. The most common eye disease caused by *diabetes*.

dialysis   A technique used to filter waste products from the blood when *kidney* function is impaired.

dilation and curettage   See *D and C*.

diuretic   An *antihypertensive* that rids the body of excess water or salt by increasing the amount lost in urine.

diverticula   Small bulges or pouches protruding through the intestinal wall that can also develop in the esophagus and *urethra*.

diverticulitis   Inflammation or infection of *diverticula*.

diverticulosis   The presence of *diverticula* in the intestines.

DNA   Deoxyribonucleic acid. The molecular structure inside every cell that carries genetic information.

do-not-resuscitate order   An *advance directive* that states that no one should perform heroic measures, including *CPR* and the use of mechanical life-support equipment, to restart a person's heart should it stop.

durable power of attorney for healthcare   An *advance directive* in which a competent person gives another person the power to make healthcare decisions on his or her behalf.

dysthymia   A chronic, less intense form of *depression*.

E

ECG   Electrocardiography. A procedure used to examine the electrical activity of the heart. The information recorded during the procedure is called an electrocardiogram.

echocardiography   An *ultrasound* examination of the heart. The information recorded during the procedure is called an echocardiogram.

E coli infection   A potentially fatal form of *food poisoning* caused by the bacterium Escherichia coli. Usually results from eating contaminated ground beef but other sources include unpasteurized dairy products and unpasteurized fruit juice.

eczema, atopic   A recurrent, inflammatory skin condition that tends to run in families and produces redness, itching, and scaly patches.

edema   Abnormal accumulation of fluid in the body tissues.

EEG   Electroencephalography. An examination of the electrical activity of the brain. The information recorded during the procedure is called an electroencephalogram.

electrocardiography   See *ECG*.

electroencephalography   See *EEG*.

electrolytes   *Sodium, potassium*, and other essential minerals that are involved in regulating various body processes.

embolism   Interruption of blood flow in a blood vessel by an *embolus*.

embolus   A plug of material (such as a *blood clot* or an air bubble) that can travel in the bloodstream and block a blood vessel.

emphysema   A disease in which the tiny air sacs in the lungs become damaged, causing chronic shortness of breath. Usually results from smoking and sometimes leads to respiratory failure or *heart failure*.

encephalitis   Inflammation of the brain, often caused by a viral infection.

endocrine system   A network of glands, organs, and tissues that produce and secrete *hormones* directly into the bloodstream to regulate many essential body processes.

endocrine therapy   See *hormone therapy*.

endometriosis   A common condition in which cells similar to those that normally line the uterus grow outside the uterus, on or near the fallopian tubes or ovaries, or in other areas of the abdominal cavity.

endorphins   Chemicals in the brain that can improve mood and help control a person's response to pain and stress.

endoscopy   A procedure that uses a lighted viewing instrument called an endoscope to look inside a body cavity or organ to diagnose or treat disorders.

enzyme   A *protein* that controls chemical reactions in the body.

epicondylitis   Inflammation of the *tendons* that attach the forearm muscles to the elbow, usually caused by *repetitive stress injury* of the forearm. Golfer's elbow and tennis elbow are two types of epicondylitis.

epidural anesthesia   A method of pain relief in which an anesthetic is injected into the area surrounding the spinal cord, blocking the nerves that lead to the chest and lower half of the body.

epilepsy   A condition characterized by recurrent *seizures* caused by abnormal electrical activity in the brain.

epinephrine   Also called adrenaline. A *hormone* produced by the *adrenal glands* that increases *heart rate* and blood flow and improves breathing.

Epstein-Barr virus   A *herpesvirus* that causes *mononucleosis*.

ERCP   Endoscopic retrograde cholangiopancreatography. An X-ray procedure that uses *endoscopy* and a *contrast medium* to examine the *gallbladder, bile* ducts, and *pancreas*.

erectile dysfunction   Formerly called impotence. The persistent inability to achieve and maintain an erection sufficient to complete sexual intercourse.

essential hypertension   See *primary hypertension.*

estrogen   Any of a group of *hormones* secreted by the ovaries that are essential for normal female sexual development and for the healthy functioning of the female reproductive system.

F

fecal occult blood   See *occult blood.*

fetal alcohol syndrome   A group of birth defects that result from excessive alcohol consumption by a pregnant woman. The most common preventable cause of mental retardation in the United States.

fiber   The indigestible nutrient found in fruits and vegetables that passes through the digestive tract without being absorbed, provides bulk to help the digestive tract function properly, and may help prevent *colon* cancer.

fibrillation   Recurrent, inefficient contraction of a muscle, especially the heart muscle.

fibroid   A noncancerous tumor of muscle and *connective tissue* growing in the wall of the uterus.

folic acid   A B vitamin essential for cell growth and repair and for production of red blood cells. Taking 400 micrograms daily during pregnancy helps prevent *neural tube defects.*

food poisoning   An adverse reaction to consuming food or drink that is contaminated with microorganisms such as bacteria or viruses. Common symptoms include diarrhea, abdominal pain, and nausea and vomiting. See individual entries: *botulism, campylobacter poisoning, coccidian infection, E coli infection, salmonella poisoning, shigella poisoning,* and s*taphylococcus poisoning.*

free radicals   Molecules produced in the body (by normal cell activity or by external agents such as radiation and cigarette smoke) that change, damage, or break down cells and are a major cause of disease and aging.

G

gallbladder   A small, pear-shaped, muscular sac under the right lobe of the *liver* that stores *bile* until the bile is needed for digestion.

gallstone   A small, hardened mass composed of *cholesterol, calcium* salts, and *bile* pigments (any of the coloring matters of bile). Can form in the *gallbladder* or in a bile duct.

gastroesophageal reflux disease   See *GERD.*

gastrointestinal series   See *GI series.*

gene   The portion of the *DNA* molecule that is the basic functional unit of heredity (the transmission of characteristics from parents to children). Contains instructions to make one or more proteins.

generalized anxiety disorder   A mental disorder characterized by persistent, unrealistic worry or fear about common occurrences such as work, health, and family relationships.

genetics   The branch of biology that deals with heredity (the transmission of characteristics from parents to children).

genitourinary tract   The organs concerned with sexual reproduction and with producing and excreting urine.

genomics   The study of *genes* and their function. Has an essential role in understanding and diagnosing disease, developing new medications, and advancing gene therapy (treatment of genetic diseases by supplementing or replacing defective genes with healthy genes).

GERD   Gastroesophageal reflux disease. A digestive disorder in which the valve connecting the esophagus and stomach does not close properly, allowing stomach acids and other irritants to flow backward into the esophagus.

GI series   Gastrointestinal series. Diagnostic procedures in which a series of X rays of the digestive tract are taken after a person swallows a barium mixture or receives a barium enema.

glaucoma   Abnormally high pressure inside the eyeball that damages peripheral (side) vision, causing the visual field to become increasingly narrow until total blindness occurs.

glucose   A simple sugar that is the body's main source of energy.

glucose meter   A device used by people with *diabetes* to measure blood *glucose* levels.

golfer's elbow   See *epicondylitis*.

gonorrhea   A common *sexually transmitted disease* caused by the gonococcus bacterium. Women often have no symptoms or mild symptoms. When symptoms occur, men and women may have burning or itching during urination and a puslike discharge from the *urethra* (in addition, women may have a vaginal discharge).

gout   A metabolic disorder characterized by high levels of uric acid in the blood, causing *joint* pain and inflammation, usually in a single joint.

granuloma   A tumorlike mass of cells.

Graves' disease   An *autoimmune disease* in which an overactive *thyroid gland* produces too much thyroid *hormone*. Symptoms include weight loss, an enlarged thyroid gland, and bulging eyes.

H

hay fever   Also called allergic rhinitis. An *allergic reaction* that causes inflammation of the *mucous membrane* lining the nose. Symptoms include coughing, stuffy nose, and sneezing.

headache   There are three main types of headache. A tension, or muscle contraction, headache is the most common type, characterized by mild to moderate pain in the head or neck and muscle tenderness. A cluster headache is a series of recurring headaches that affects one side of the head and usually includes symptoms such as a runny nose and watery eyes. A migraine is a severe, persistent, sometimes disabling headache that occurs on one side of the head but may spread to the other side and can be accompanied by nausea, vomiting, sensitivity to light and noise, fever, chills, aches, and sweating.

heart attack   Also called myocardial infarction (MI). Sudden death of a section of the heart muscle caused by a loss of blood supply. The most common cause is blockage of blood flow in one of the coronary *arteries* by a *thrombus*. Symptoms include severe, constant chest pain; shortness of breath; nausea; vomiting; restlessness; cold, clammy skin; and loss of consciousness. Risk factors include *atherosclerosis*, obesity, *diabetes*, *high blood pressure*, and a high blood level of *cholesterol*.

heartbeat   Contraction of the heart muscle that pumps blood into the *arteries* and throughout the body.

heart disease   Also called coronary artery disease. A condition in which one or more coronary *arteries* become narrowed or blocked, reducing or cutting off blood flow to the heart muscle, and damaging the heart.

heart failure   The inability of the heart to pump blood efficiently, leading to congestion of blood in *veins* and excessive accumulation of fluid in body tissues.

heart rate   The number of *heartbeats* per minute.

hematuria   The presence of red blood cells in the urine.

hemochromatosis   A hereditary metabolic disorder in which excessive amounts of iron accumulate in body tissues, potentially damaging them.

hemodialysis   A form of *dialysis* in which blood circulates through a machine where it is filtered and purified before being returned to the body. Used to treat *kidney* failure.

hemoglobin   The oxygen-carrying *protein* in red blood cells.

hepatitis   Inflammation of the *liver* that may be caused by infection, drugs, or toxins.

hernia   Protrusion of a portion of an organ or tissue through a weak area in the muscle wall that normally contains it.

herniated disk   See *prolapsed disk*.

herpes, genital   A *sexually transmitted disease* caused by herpes simplex virus 2 and characterized by recurrent outbreaks of small, red, painful blisters on the genital area, buttocks, anus, or thighs. Can be spread to another person between outbreaks even if the infected person is symptom-free. Has no known cure.

herpes simplex virus 1   A *herpesvirus* that usually affects areas of the body other than the genitals.

herpes simplex virus 2　A *herpesvirus* that causes genital herpes. See *herpes, genital*.

herpesvirus　Any of a group of viruses that includes *herpes simplex virus 1, herpes simplex virus 2, varicella-zoster virus, Epstein-Barr virus,* and *cytomegalovirus*.

high-altitude pulmonary edema　A life-threatening buildup of fluid in the lungs that can result from rapid ascent to high altitudes.

high blood pressure　Also called hypertension. A condition in which *blood pressure* is persistently raised. See also *primary hypertension, pulmonary hypertension,* and *secondary hypertension*.

hip replacement　See *arthroplasty*.

histamine　A chemical released by the body during an *allergic reaction* that produces symptoms of inflammation, including redness, swelling, heat, and pain.

HIV　Human immunodeficiency virus. A virus that infects the cells of the *immune system* and causes *AIDS*. Transmitted primarily through contact with an infected person's blood, semen, or vaginal or anal secretions; can also be transmitted to a nursing baby through breast milk.

Holter monitor　A portable device worn around the neck or over the shoulder that records the electrical activity of the heart during a 24-hour period.

homocysteine　A body chemical that at an elevated level increases the risk of *heart disease*. Taking 400 micrograms of the B vitamin *folic acid* every day helps keep homocysteine at a healthy level.

hormone replacement therapy　The use of synthetic or natural *hormones* to treat a disease, disorder, or hormone deficiency. For example, the female hormones *estrogen* and *progesterone* are used to relieve symptoms of menopause.

hormones　Chemicals, such as *insulin*, that are produced by the body and released directly into the bloodstream to perform specific functions.

hormone therapy　Also called endocrine therapy. Treatment of a disease such as cancer using *hormones* that affect the growth of cells in the body.

hospice　A program that provides comfort and care to dying people in their own home or sometimes in a hospital or nursing home setting. Emphasizes quality of life and focuses on relieving pain and controlling other symptoms.

HPV　Human papillomavirus. Any of a number of strains of viruses that cause *warts*. In women, HPV is the most common cause of cervical cancer; in men, it increases the risk of cancer of the penis.

HRT　See *hormone replacement therapy*.

human immunodeficiency virus　See *HIV*.

human papillomavirus　See *HPV*.

hydrogenated fats   Vegetable oils that have been converted into a solid form such as stick margarine or canned shortening. Can raise the level of harmful low-density lipoprotein *cholesterol* in the blood.

hyperglycemia   An abnormally high level of *glucose* in the blood. Usually occurs in people with untreated or improperly regulated *diabetes*.

hypertension   See *high blood pressure*. See also *primary hypertension, pulmonary hypertension*, and *secondary hypertension*.

hypoglycemia   An abnormally low level of *glucose* in the blood. Usually occurs when a person with *diabetes* takes too much *insulin* or misses a meal but can also occur in people who do not have diabetes.

hypothalamus   A small structure at the base of the brain that regulates many body functions, including appetite and body temperature.

I

ileostomy   A surgical procedure in which the ileum (the longest, narrowest part of the small intestine) is brought through an incision in the abdominal wall and an artificial opening is created through which feces can be discharged into a bag attached to the skin.

immune system   A network of specialized cells and organs that protects the body from infectious organisms and from cancer.

immunization   The process of activating the *immune system* to protect against a specific infectious organism. Performed by injecting *antibodies* into the bloodstream or by stimulating the immune system to produce its own antibodies.

immunodeficiency   Impaired effectiveness of the *immune system*.

immunoglobulins   See *antibodies*.

immunotherapy   Treatment to stimulate the *immune system* to destroy cancer cells.

impotence   See *erectile dysfunction*.

incontinence   Urinary incontinence is the involuntary leaking of urine during activities (such as coughing, sneezing, or jogging) that increase pressure inside the abdomen. Fecal incontinence is the inability to control bowel movements.

inflammatory bowel disease   A term that refers to either of two chronic disorders of the intestine—*ulcerative colitis* or *Crohn's disease*.

insulin   A *hormone* produced by the *pancreas* that is essential for the body's use of *glucose* for energy.

intracerebral hemorrhage   Bleeding from a ruptured blood vessel into the tissues of the brain. See also *stroke*.

intravenous pyelogram   See *urography, intravenous*.

in vitro fertilization   A method of treating infertility in which an egg is removed from a woman, fertilized in the laboratory, and reinserted into her uterus or a fallopian tube.

irritable bowel syndrome   An intestinal disorder characterized by recurrent abdominal pain and bouts of diarrhea or constipation. Occurs in otherwise healthy adults and usually is associated with stress.

ischemia   A temporary decrease in the supply of oxygen to an organ or tissue.

IVP   Intravenous pyelogram. See *urography, intravenous*.

J

jaundice   Yellowing of the skin and the whites of the eyes.

jock itch   Also called tinea cruris. A common, contagious, fungal infection that produces red, itchy, irritated skin in the groin area, inner thighs, or around the anus.

joint   A point at which two or more bones meet; most joints allow movement.

joint replacement   See *arthroplasty*.

K

Kaposi's sarcoma   A type of skin cancer characterized by small, reddish-purple tumors that first appear on the feet and ankles and later spread to other parts of the body. Primarily affects people with *AIDS*.

keratin   A tough, fibrous *protein* in skin, hair, and nails.

kidney   One of a pair of abdominal organs that filter waste products and excess water from the blood and have an essential role in maintaining *blood pressure*.

kidney stone   A small, hard mass of mineral salts that can form in a *kidney*.

knee replacement   See *arthroplasty*.

L

lactase   An *enzyme* needed to break down *lactose* during digestion.

lactose   One of the sugars found in milk. Lactose intolerance is the inability to digest lactose due to a deficiency of *lactase*.

laparoscopy   Examination of or surgery in the abdomen using a viewing tube called a laparoscope and special instruments inserted through tiny incisions in the abdomen.

LASIK   Laser in situ keratolileusis. A surgical procedure in which a doctor uses a laser to reshape the *cornea* to correct nearsightedness, farsightedness, or astigmatism.

Legionnaires' disease   A form of *pneumonia* caused by a bacterium that contaminates water and air-conditioning systems.

leukemia   Any of various forms of cancer characterized by abnormal proliferation and production of white blood cells in the bone marrow.

libido   Sexual desire.

ligament   Tough, fibrous tissue that connects bone to bone and provides stability in a *joint*.

light therapy   See *phototherapy*.

lithotripsy   A procedure that uses ultrasonic shock waves to break up stones (such as *kidney stones*) that have formed in the urinary tract.

liver   An abdominal organ that produces chemicals needed by the body and controls the levels of many chemicals in the blood.

living will   An *advance directive* prepared by a competent person that indicates his or her wishes regarding life-sustaining medical treatments. Goes into effect after the person is unable to speak for himself or herself and can be revised or withdrawn by the person at any time.

Lou Gehrig's disease   See *ALS*.

lumbar puncture   A diagnostic procedure in which a hollow needle is used to remove cerebrospinal fluid from the lower part of the spinal canal for testing.

lumpectomy   A surgical procedure for breast cancer in which the tumor and a small amount of surrounding tissue are removed. Usually some lymph nodes from under the arm also are removed to determine whether the cancer has spread.

lupus   A chronic *autoimmune disease* that affects *connective tissue* and numerous organs and can cause inflammation in any part of the body, including the skin, *joints*, heart, lungs, *kidneys*, nervous system, and blood. More common in women than in men.

luteinizing hormone   A *hormone* produced in the *pituitary gland* that helps regulate the menstrual cycle in women and the production of sperm in men.

Lyme disease   A bacterial infection transmitted by a tick bite that causes a rash, fever, and inflammation of the *joints* and the heart.

lymph nodes   Small glands clustered in the neck, armpits, abdomen, and groin that are part of the body's *immune system*. Supply infection-fighting cells to the bloodstream and filter out bacteria and other substances that stimulate the production of *antibodies*.

lymphocyte   A specialized white blood cell that protects the body from invading microorganisms and cancer cells. Two types are B lymphocytes (B cells) and T lymphocytes (T cells).

lymphoma   Any of a group of cancers of the lymphatic system that can occur in any part of the body and can spread.

M

macula   The part of the *retina* that provides sharp sight in the center of the field of vision and is essential for seeing fine detail.

macular degeneration   Age-related damage to the *macula*. Macular degeneration is the leading cause of blindness in people over 50.

magnetic resonance imaging   See *MRI*.

malignant   Cancerous.

mammography   An X-ray procedure used to detect breast cancer at an early stage. The X-ray image produced during this procedure is called a mammogram.

manic-depressive disorder   See *bipolar disorder.*

melanin   The pigment that gives skin, hair, and eyes their color.

melanoma, malignant   The most serious form of skin cancer, the first sign of which is often a change in an existing *mole*. Spreads quickly and can be fatal. Usually results from overexposure to sunlight.

melatonin   A *hormone* produced in the brain that regulates the sleep-wake cycle.

Ménière's disease   An inner-ear disorder characterized by dizziness, loss of balance, *tinnitus*, and hearing loss.

meningitis   Inflammation of the meninges (the membranes surrounding the brain and spinal cord), usually as the result of infection.

metabolism   The chemical processes that take place in the body.

metastasis   The spread of cancer from its original location to another location in the body.

MI   Myocardial infarction. See *heart attack*.

ministroke   See *TIA*.

minoxidil   An *antihypertensive* that is also available in nonprescription lotion form to treat male pattern baldness.

mitral valve   The valve in the heart that allows blood to flow from the left *atrium* to the left *ventricle*.

mitral valve prolapse   A common, usually minor defect of the *mitral valve* in which the valve does not close properly, allowing small amounts of blood to leak back into the left *atrium* from the left *ventricle*.

mitral valve regurgitation   Also called mitral incompetence or mitral insufficiency. Leakage of blood back through the *mitral valve* into the left *atrium* each time the left *ventricle* contracts, leading to increased *blood pressure* in the blood vessels from the lungs to the heart.

mitral valve stenosis   A narrowing of the *mitral valve* opening that increases resistance to blood flow from the left *atrium* to the left *ventricle*. Can eventually lead to *heart failure*.

mole   A dark-colored growth on the skin that may be flat or raised and that may vary in size. Moles can appear anywhere on the body. In rare cases, a mole may develop into a serious form of skin cancer called malignant melanoma (see *melanoma, malignant*).

molluscum contagiosum   A common, harmless viral infection characterized by tiny lumps on the skin that is often transmitted sexually and usually clears up without treatment in a few months.

mononucleosis   An infectious disease caused by the Epstein-Barr virus and characterized by fever, sore throat, and swollen glands.

monounsaturated fat   A type of *unsaturated fat*—found in olive oil, canola oil, and peanut oil—that lowers total *cholesterol* and harmful low-density lipoprotein *cholesterol.*

motor neuron disease   A group of rare disorders characterized by degeneration of nerves that control muscle activity in the brain and spinal cord, resulting in weakness and wasting of the muscles. Of unknown cause. See also *Parkinson's disease.*

MRI   Magnetic resonance imaging. A diagnostic technique that uses a computer, a powerful magnetic field, and radio waves to produce detailed two- and three-dimensional images of body tissues that are displayed on a video monitor.

MS   Multiple sclerosis. A progressive, disabling disorder characterized by degeneration of the protective coverings of nerve cells.

mucous membrane   The thin, skinlike lining of the cavities and tubes in the body, such as the digestive tract, urinary tract, and respiratory tract.

mucus   A thick, slimy fluid secreted by a *mucous membrane* to lubricate and protect the part of the body that it lines.

multiple sclerosis   See *MS.*

myelography   A diagnostic examination in which a *contrast medium* is injected and X rays are taken of the spinal cord, nerves, and other tissues in and around the spinal canal. The information recorded during the procedure is called a myelogram.

myocardial infarction   See *heart attack.*

N

neural tube defects   Birth defects that result from failure of the brain or spinal cord to develop normally in an embryo.

neuron   A nerve cell.

neurotransmitters   Chemicals in the brain that enable brain cells to communicate with each other.

nongonococcal urethritis   A common *sexually transmitted disease* that is usually caused by a *chlamydia* infection. Symptoms in both men and women include pain during urination and a discharge of mucus from the *urethra.*

nonsteroidal anti-inflammatory drugs   See *NSAIDs.*

noradrenaline   See *norepinephrine.*

norepinephrine   Also called noradrenaline. A *hormone* that helps regulate *heart rate* and *blood pressure* by narrowing blood vessels and increasing heart rate when blood pressure drops below the normal level.

NSAIDs   Nonsteroidal anti-inflammatory drugs. Medications such as ibuprofen and naproxen that relieve pain and inflammation.

O

obsessive-compulsive disorder   A mental disorder characterized by persistent thoughts or impulses (obsessions) that lead to repetitive, ritualized thoughts or behaviors (compulsions).

occult blood   The presence of blood in body fluids or in feces that cannot be seen by the naked eye but can be detected by chemical tests. Occult blood tests are used to screen for cancer and to diagnose various disorders of the digestive tract.

opportunistic infections   Infections that rarely occur in healthy people but frequently occur in people who have impaired *immune systems* such as people with *AIDS.*

optic nerve   One of a pair of nerves that transmit information about visual images.

osteoarthritis   Progressive, gradual thinning or destruction of *cartilage* in the *joints,* usually resulting from aging, injury, or overuse.

osteomalacia   Softening, weakening, and loss of minerals from the bones of an adult resulting from a deficiency of vitamin D.

osteoporosis   A disorder in which bones become thin, brittle, and more susceptible to fracture. Although osteoporosis is more common in women, it also can occur in men.

otolaryngologist   A physician who specializes in treating disorders of the ear, nose, and throat.

oxidation   A damaging chemical reaction in body cells caused by the actions of *free radicals.*

oxygen free radicals   See *free radicals.*

P

pacemaker   An electronic device implanted in the chest to regulate the *heartbeat.*

palpitations   An unusually strong, rapid *heartbeat.*

pancreas   A long, irregularly shaped gland behind the stomach that secretes digestive *enzymes* and *hormones* such as *insulin.*

pancreatitis   Inflammation of the *pancreas* that can result from alcohol abuse, *gallstones,* injury to the abdomen, or use of some medications.

panic disorder   A mental disorder characterized by brief, intense episodes of high anxiety (called panic attacks) that occur for no apparent reason.

Pap smear   A diagnostic test in which cells are scraped from the surface of the cervix and examined under a microscope to detect abnormal cells that are or could become cancerous.

parathyroid glands   Two pairs of glands located near the *thyroid gland* in the neck. Produce parathyroid *hormone*, which helps control the level of *calcium* in the blood.

Parkinson's disease   A *motor neuron disease* most common in people over age 60 that causes weakness, rigidity, and *tremors* in the muscles.

peak-flow meter   An instrument used to evaluate the severity of *asthma* by measuring the highest rate at which a person can exhale.

pelvis   The basin-shaped bony structure at the base of the spine, consisting of the ilium (part of the hipbone), the sacrum, and the coccyx (tailbone). Protects organs such as the bladder and rectum.

pericarditis   Inflammation of the pericardium (the membrane that surrounds the heart) that often leads to chest pain and fever.

peripheral vascular disease   Poor circulation in the legs, and sometimes in the arms, caused by narrowing of blood vessels in the affected area.

peritoneum   The membrane that lines the abdominal cavity and covers the abdominal organs.

peritonitis   Inflammation of the *peritoneum*, usually as a result of a bacterial infection in the abdominal cavity.

PET scan   Positron emission tomography scan. A computerized, diagnostic imaging technique that produces two- or three-dimensional images that show the function of tissues such as those of the brain, heart, and blood vessels.

phlebitis   Also called thrombophlebitis. Inflammation and *thrombus* formation in a *vein*, usually in the legs.

phobia   Persistent, irrational anxiety about a particular object, person, place, or situation.

phototherapy   Also called light therapy. Uses ultraviolet light to treat a form of *depression* called *seasonal affective disorder* and skin disorders such as acne and *psoriasis*.

pituitary gland   A gland at the base of the brain that secretes *hormones* and regulates and controls other hormone-secreting glands and many body processes, including reproduction.

plaque, arterial   Fatty material that builds up inside *artery* walls. Can eventually lead to *atherosclerosis*.

plaque, dental   A sticky coating of saliva, bacteria, and food debris that forms on the teeth.

pleura   See *pleural membranes*.

pleural membranes Two membranes that line the chest cavity and cover the lungs.

pleurisy Inflammation of the *pleural membranes*, usually caused by a lung infection. Causes chest pain that may travel to the shoulder on the affected side.

pneumonia Inflammation of the lungs, usually caused by a viral or bacterial infection. Symptoms include fever, chills, shortness of breath, and coughing up blood or yellow-green sputum.

polyp A growth that projects, usually on a stalk, from a body membrane. Can develop into cancer.

polyunsaturated fat A type of *unsaturated fat*—found in safflower, sunflower, soy bean, corn, and cottonseed oil—that lowers total *cholesterol* and the beneficial high-density lipoprotein cholesterol.

posttraumatic stress disorder A persistent disturbance of emotions and behavior that develops after experiencing extreme trauma, such as being a victim of or witnessing a violent crime or participating in military combat.

potassium An essential mineral that helps the body maintain water balance, conduct nerve signals, contract muscles, and maintain a normal *heartbeat*.

primary hypertension Also called essential hypertension. *High blood pressure* of unknown cause.

proctoscopy Examination of the anus and rectum with a viewing tube.

progesterone A female sex *hormone* produced by the ovaries that is essential for a healthy pregnancy. Ensures healthy development of the fetus by promoting normal growth and functioning of the placenta.

prolapsed disk Also called a herniated disk. A disorder in which one of the pads of *cartilage* between the vertebrae of the spine protrudes and presses on a *ligament* or nerve, causing back pain.

prostaglandins Substances similar to *hormones* that occur in many body tissues and produce a variety of effects throughout the body, such as pain and inflammation in damaged tissue.

prostatectomy Surgical removal of all or part of the *prostate gland*.

prostate gland The gland that secretes a fluid that is a major component of semen.

prostate-specific antigen See *PSA*.

prostatitis Inflammation of the *prostate gland* usually caused by a bacterial infection.

proteins Complex substances composed of *amino acids* that form the structure of all living matter.

PSA Prostate-specific antigen. A *protein* produced by the *prostate gland*. Because PSA is not normally found in blood, high levels of the protein in blood can indicate prostate cancer but can also indicate less serious problems such as an enlarged prostate gland. A PSA test measures the levels of PSA in the blood.

psoriasis A common, chronic skin disorder characterized by red, dry, itchy patches of skin with silvery scales. Most often affects the scalp, nails, arms, legs, groin, and lower back.

psychotherapy Describes a variety of treatments for mental or emotional disorders. Used to help people change their behavior through techniques such as talking, reinforcement, reassurance, and support.

pulmonary embolism A life-threatening condition that occurs when a *blood clot* forms in a *vein*, travels through the bloodstream, and blocks an *artery* in the lung.

pulmonary hypertension *High blood pressure* in the *arteries* that supply blood to the lungs.

pulmonary rehabilitation Comprehensive, multidisciplinary therapy to improve the comfort and functioning of a person who has chronic lung disease.

pulse The rhythmic expansion and contraction of an *artery* as blood is pumped through it.

PUVA Psoralen and ultraviolet A. A treatment that combines the use of psoralens (drugs that make the skin sensitive to light) and ultraviolet light to treat skin conditions such as *psoriasis*.

pyelogram, intravenous See *urography, intravenous*.

pyelonephritis Inflammation of a *kidney*, usually caused by a bacterial infection.

R

radiation therapy Also called radiotherapy. Treatment using X rays or other forms of radiation to destroy or slow the spread of cancer cells.

radioallergosorbent test See *RAST*.

radionuclide scanning A diagnostic imaging technique in which a radioactive substance that is swallowed or injected into the bloodstream collects in a target organ, allowing a camera to produce images of the organ.

RAST Radioallergosorbent test. A test that detects *antibodies* to specific *allergens*. Used to diagnose *allergies*.

rectal examination, digital An examination in which a doctor inserts a lubricated, gloved finger into a person's rectum and feels for abnormalities in the abdomen or pelvis or in the *prostate gland* in men or ovaries in women. The examination is also performed to look for *occult blood* and to evaluate the rectum.

remission A partial or complete disappearance of the signs and symptoms of a disorder or disease.

repetitive stress injury   Also called repetitive strain injury. An injury caused by persistent repetition of the same movement.

rest, ice, compression, and elevation   See *RICE*.

restless legs syndrome   A sleep disorder characterized by unpleasant sensations in the legs.

retina   The light-sensitive membrane that lines the inside of the back of the eye.

retinoids   Vitamin A–like medications that are used to treat skin conditions such as acne and *psoriasis*.

Reye's syndrome   A rare, life-threatening disorder that causes a child's brain and liver to swell after a viral infection such as the flu, chickenpox, or a cold. Has been linked to aspirin and other salicylate-containing medications used to treat viral infections.

rheumatoid arthritis   A chronic, *autoimmune disease* that causes pain, swelling, and stiffness in the affected *joints*. In severe cases the joints are completely destroyed. Also can affect the heart, lungs, and eyes.

RICE   Rest, ice, compression, and elevation. Standard self-treatment for most *strains*, *sprains*, and muscle pulls.

rickets   A nutritional deficiency caused by a lack of vitamin D that leads to weakening and softening of the bones, usually in the legs.

rosacea   A chronic, acnelike skin disorder in adults marked by an abnormally red nose and red cheeks. Of unknown cause.

rotator cuff   The arrangement of muscles and *tendons* surrounding the shoulder *joint* and providing movement and stability.

S

SAD   See *seasonal affective disorder*.

salmonella poisoning   A form of *food poisoning* from eating food such as eggs, milk, raw meat, raw poultry, or raw fish that is contaminated with salmonella bacteria. Can be very serious in infants, young children, older people, and people who are chronically ill or whose *immune systems* are weakened.

saturated fat   A type of fat in the diet, found in dairy products and meat, that can raise the level of *cholesterol* in the blood and increase the risk of *heart disease* and some forms of cancer. See also *unsaturated fat*.

schizophrenia   A serious, disabling mental disorder characterized by distorted thoughts, emotions, and behavior.

sclerotherapy   A procedure for treating *varicose veins* in which an irritant solution is injected into an affected vein, causing its walls to stick together and block the flow of blood through the vein. Nearby veins then take over the work of the treated vein.

seasonal affective disorder   A form of *depression* that tends to occur during the fall and winter, when there are fewer hours of sunlight.

secondary hypertension   *High blood pressure* that can be cured by treating its underlying cause.

seizure   Excessive electrical activity in the brain that causes temporary loss of consciousness, memory, or movement. See also *epilepsy*.

sensorineural hearing loss   Deafness caused by damage to the inner ear or a nerve. May result from a congenital defect, disease, or trauma.

serotonin   A substance present in the brain and other body tissues that acts as a *neurotransmitter* and is involved in regulating mood.

sexually transmitted disease   An infection transmitted primarily through sexual contact (genital, oral, or anal) with an infected person.

shigella poisoning   A highly infectious form of *food poisoning* that usually occurs in people who have been exposed to food—such as raw vegetables; dairy products; or potato, tuna, chicken, or macaroni salads—or water that is contaminated with shigella bacteria.

shingles   Infection of the nerves that supply the skin, resulting in a painful rash of small, crusting blisters. Caused by the same virus that causes chickenpox and occurs only in people who have had chickenpox or who have been exposed to the virus.

shin splints   Pain in the front and sides of the lower part of the legs caused by *strain* or damage to underlying structures. Can worsen during exercise.

sickle-cell disease   Also called sickle-cell anemia. An inherited blood disorder characterized by deformed, sickle-shaped red blood cells that contain an abnormal form of *hemoglobin*. These fragile blood cells break up easily, blocking and damaging blood vessels and reducing the supply of oxygen to organs and tissues.

SIDS   Sudden infant death syndrome. The sudden, unexpected death of a previously healthy infant during sleep. Putting a child to sleep on his or her back or side reduces the risk.

sigmoidoscopy   Examination of the rectum and sigmoid *colon* (the lower part of the colon) using a viewing instrument called a sigmoidoscope that is passed into the body through the anus.

sinoatrial node   The heart's internal pacemaker, which sends out electrical impulses that tell the heart when to contract.

sleep apnea   A potentially life-threatening sleep disorder characterized by brief, involuntary interruptions of breathing during sleep.

sodium   An essential mineral (salt) that helps the body maintain water balance and *blood pressure*.

SPF   Sun protection factor. A number assigned to a *sunscreen* that indicates the level of protection it provides from the sun's damaging ultraviolet rays. The higher the number, the greater the level of protection. Doctors recommend that people use a sunscreen with an SPF of 15 or greater.

sphygmomanometer   An instrument—made up of an inflatable cuff, a rubber bulb, and a gauge, glass column, or digital readout display—used to measure *blood pressure.*

spirometry　A test that measures the volume of air entering and leaving the lungs. Performed to diagnose or monitor lung disorders. The instrument used to perform the test is called a spirometer.

sprain　Stretching or tearing of *ligaments* in a *joint.*

squamous cell carcinoma　A common type of skin cancer (most common in light-skinned, fair-haired people over 60) that develops in cells on the surface of the skin. Usually caused by long-term overexposure to sunlight.

staphylococcus poisoning　A form of *food poisoning* that usually occurs after eating food such as meat, poultry, eggs, milk, cream-filled bakery goods, tuna salad, or potato salad that has not been properly refrigerated.

STD　See *sexually transmitted disease.*

stenosis　Narrowing of a duct, canal, body passage, or tubular organ. See also *aortic stenosis* and *mitral valve stenosis.*

stent　A tiny device made of metallic or plastic wire mesh that is used to keep an *artery* open after *angioplasty.*

steroids　See *corticosteroids.*

stoma　A surgically constructed opening, especially in the abdominal wall.

strain　Stretching or tearing of *tendons* and their attached muscles.

strep throat　A throat infection caused by *streptococcus.* Symptoms include sore throat, fever, and enlarged lymph nodes in the neck.

streptococcus　A common type of spherical bacterium that normally lives on the skin and in the mouth, throat, and intestines.

stress fracture　A fracture caused by repeated trauma or overuse of a bone.

stroke　Also called a cerebrovascular accident. Sudden damage to part of the brain caused by an interruption in blood flow to the area. Ischemic stroke, the most common type, results from blockage of a blood vessel in the brain. Hemorrhagic stroke results from a ruptured blood vessel in the brain. See also *intracerebral hemorrhage* and *TIA.*

sudden infant death syndrome　See *SIDS.*

sun protection factor　See *SPF.*

sunscreensz　Preparations applied to the skin that help protect it from the damaging ultraviolet rays in sunlight.

syphilis　A *sexually transmitted disease* caused by infection with a bacterium that enters the body through broken skin or through the *mucous membranes* in the genitals, rectum, or mouth. Can cause serious damage to tissues and organs throughout the body if untreated.

T

tachycardia　An unusually rapid *heart rate* of more than 100 beats per minute.

temporomandibular disorder   See *TMD.*

tendinitis   Inflammation of a *tendon,* usually caused by excess friction between a tendon and a bone.

tendon   Strong, fibrous tissue that connects muscle to bone.

tennis elbow   See *epicondylitis.*

testosterone   The key male sex *hormone,* which stimulates muscle growth and the development of male sex characteristics.

thrombolytics   Medications used to dissolve *blood clots* in cases of *embolism, thrombosis,* and *heart attack.*

thrombophlebitis   See *phlebitis.*

thrombosis   Formation of a *blood clot* inside a blood vessel.

thrombus   A *blood clot* that forms inside a blood vessel. A blood clot that breaks off and travels through the bloodstream is called an *embolus.*

thrush   See *candidiasis.*

thyroid gland   A gland in the neck that secretes *hormones* essential to the regulation of various body processes, including *heart rate* and *blood pressure.*

TIA   Transient ischemic attack. Also called a ministroke. A brief interruption in blood flow to the brain, causing temporary symptoms such as impaired vision, sensation, movement, or speech. See also *stroke.*

tinea cruris   See *jock itch.*

tinea pedis   See *athlete's foot.*

tinnitus   A common ear disorder characterized by persistent ringing, hissing, or other sounds in the ear that have no external source.

tissue plasminogen activator   See *TPA.*

TMD   Temporomandibular disorder. A term used to describe a painful group of disorders that affect the jaw *joints* and their supporting muscles and *ligaments.*

TPA   Tissue plasminogen activator. A *thrombolytic* used in the treatment of ischemic *stroke.*

trans fatty acids   Synthetic fats produced during food processing.

transient ischemic attack   See *TIA.*

tremor   Involuntary, rhythmic muscle movement—most often in the hands, feet, jaw, tongue, or head—caused by alternating contraction and relaxation of the muscles.

trichomoniasis   A common *sexually transmitted disease* that often causes no symptoms. When symptoms occur, men and women may have pain during urination. Women may also have a yellow-green vaginal discharge with an unpleasant odor; men may have a clear discharge from the penis.

triglycerides   The major fats in the blood. A high level of triglycerides indicates an increased risk of *heart disease, high blood pressure,* and *diabetes.*

tubal ligation   A sterilization procedure in which a woman's fallopian tubes are surgically sealed or cut.

U

ulcer   An open sore on the skin or on a *mucous membrane*. A peptic ulcer is a hole or break in the lining of the stomach or duodenum (the first section of the small intestine) that is usually caused by a type of bacterium but in rare cases can be caused by excess stomach acid.

ulcerative colitis   Chronic ulceration and inflammation of the lining of the *mucous membrane* of the *colon* and rectum.

ultrasound   A diagnostic imaging procedure that uses high-frequency sound waves to create a picture of internal body structures on a video screen.

unsaturated fat   A type of fat found in most vegetable oils that does not raise *cholesterol* levels in the blood. See individual entries: *monounsaturated fat* and *polyunsaturated fat*. See also *saturated fat*.

urea   A waste product of the breakdown of *protein* in the body.

uremia   A toxic condition characterized by excess *urea* and other waste products in the blood. Caused by *kidney* failure.

urethra   The channel through which urine is discharged from the bladder and, in males, through which semen is discharged.

urethral stricture   Narrowing or blockage of part of the male *urethra* by scar tissue from an injury or infection. Causes difficult and sometimes painful urination.

urethritis   Inflammation of the *urethra*.

urinalysis   Testing of a sample of urine for diagnostic purposes.

urography, intravenous   Also called an intravenous pyelogram (IVP). A diagnostic examination of the urinary tract in which *contrast medium* is injected into the bloodstream and X rays are taken.

V

vaccination   See *immunization*.

varicella-zoster virus   A *herpesvirus* that causes chickenpox and *shingles*.

varicose veins   Enlarged, twisted *veins* just beneath the skin that result from weakening of the valves in the veins. Most often occur in the legs.

vas deferens   One of a pair of tubes that store sperm and carry it from the testicles and epididymis (the coiled tube in which sperm mature) to the *urethra* during ejaculation.

vasectomy   A male sterilization procedure in which each *vas deferens* is cut and sealed to prevent sperm from reaching the *urethra*.

vasodilators   Medications that widen blood vessels. Used to treat such conditions as *angina* and *heart failure*.

vein   A blood vessel that carries blood from the organs and tissues to the heart.

ventricle   One of the two large lower chambers of the heart. The left ventricle is the main pumping chamber of the heart.

ventricular fibrillation   Rapid, ineffective, uncoordinated contractions of the ventricles of the heart that can be fatal if not treated immediately.

venules   Small *veins*.

W

warts   Harmless, contagious growths on the skin or *mucous membrane* caused by a viral infection. Usually appear on the feet (plantar warts), hands, or face. Genital warts (a common *sexually transmitted disease* caused by *HPV*) grow in, around, or on the reproductive organs or anus.

weight-bearing exercise   Any exercise, such as jogging, brisk walking, or stair climbing, that works the large muscles of the lower body, stimulating bone growth and building *bone density*.

Y

yeast infection   A popular term for the infection *candidiasis*.

Index